Letters to My Sisters

Plain truths and straightforward advice from a Gynecologist

Letters to My Sisters

Plain truths and straightforward advice from a Gynecologist

Claire
Best Wishes n school
Keep healthy; happy always
9/4/16

Ngozi Osuagwu, M.D., FACOG

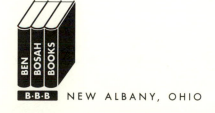

BEN BOSAH BOOKS
B·B·B NEW ALBANY, OHIO

Publisher's Cataloguing in Publication Data
Provided by Quality Books, Inc.

Osuagwu, Ngozi.
      Letters to my sisters : plain truths and
  straightforward advice from a gynecologist / Ngozi
  Osuagwu.
      Includes index.
      ISBN-13: 9780977339815
      ISBN-10: 0977339815

      1. Gynecology—Popular works. 2. Obstetrics--Popular
  works. 3. Women—Health and hygiene.   I. Title.

  RG121.O75 2006   618.1
                            QBI06-600002

Library of Congress Control Number: 2005939021

For more information about Ngozi Osuagwu, MD, FACOG
and Letters to My Sisters, visit www.letterstomysisters.com

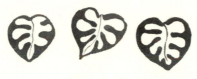

Dedication

To my parents,

Grace and Harold,

and to all my patients,

for what they have taught,

and continue to teach me.

Disclaimer

While most of the information in this book is about medical issues, it is not medical advice and should not be treated as such. The material in this book is only informational in nature, and meant to facilitate conversations with your healthcare providers. Although written by a licensed medical doctor, it is not meant as a substitute for the advice of, and care by your licensed medical professional. The letters in this book are based on the author's experience, but no references have been made to any person, nor should any be inferred. All the names are used fictitiously. The author and publisher disclaim any liability arising directly or indirectly from the use of this book.

Throughout the text, links to websites are provided. These sites were carefully screened and included correct information at the time of review; however, it is important to remember that the Internet is a dynamic entity—websites and the information posted within them are constantly changing and evolving. The information contained within these sites is not intended for diagnostic purposes, nor is it intended to replace the consultation of your own doctor or licensed medical practitioner. The author and publisher make no representation or warranty regarding the accuracy, reliability, completeness, currentness, or timeliness of the content, text, or graphics. The links provided to these websites are for information only — they do not constitute endorsements of the sites.

Acknowledgements

A book of this nature from a novice writer is never possible without lots of assistance. I want to thank the following individuals for their help in different forms and their inputs during the development of the manuscript—Crystal Adegbola, Emily Berrios, Winifred Okoye, Esq., Noreen Palmer, Dara Jackson-Wiggins, Hope Madden, Chinwe Osuagwu, Lara Lindsay, Dolvies Coke, Mary Straney and Kim Lundy. In addition to being part of the copyediting team, Kim also assisted me in selecting and annotating the websites chosen for this book. I am also grateful to Ryan Green and Fawn Veeransunthorn, who provided the medical illustrations. Lesley Ehlers made the book much better with her beautifully conceived cover, the layout of the text and the overall design of the book. I am extremely grateful to her for her patience and guidance as we worked to create this book from the manuscript.

At one point, I was one of those forty four million uninsured people in the United States. My doctors did not abandon me and thanks to their continuing care, I am alive and healthy to write this book. I am glad for the care that has been provided to me by Doctors John Blackman, Martha Brogan, Philip Hawley, Martin Kelsten, Sanford Melmed, Brenda Sickle-Santanello and last but definitely not the least, Delois Teague. They may not appear in any Best Physicians list, but to me, they are best in our profession. When a doctor is referring you to another physician, you should always find out where they would send their family members. The aforementioned individuals are among those physicians I would recommend to my own members of the family.

In January 2005, I joined the teaching staff of Doctors Hospital in Columbus. As a child of teachers, it has always been a passion of mine to also impart my knowledge to others, and the opportunity to do so was made possible by the following individuals—Kreg Gruber, Steven Bunyard, Penny Cowdery and Doctors Kirk Hilliard, Bob Falcone and

Jim Perez. To them, I am very thankful. I am also grateful for the resident physicians in the Department of Obstetrics and Gynecology, whose reviews resulted in my being given the chance to realize my dreams to teach.

Chiedu, Chidi, and Chinenye are the joys of my life and they make it complete. I am very grateful to them for all they make me and I love them dearly. To my family, immediate, nuclear, and universal, I extend my best wishes, and may the Almighty continue to bless all those who work as his instruments by bringing positive changes to the lives of many people and the world.

And how can I forget my dear Chukwuemeka, without whom I can say honestly that this book would not have been completed. I count your presence in my life and your relentless effort to always make me better personally and professionally, the best blessing bestowed on me by the Almighty.

Prologue

This book was initially conceived as a parting gift to my patients when I was contemplating leaving private practice. As with most doctors, especially those in my specialty, I was at the point of abandoning the practice of medicine because of many factors, principally declining reimbursement, increasing costs, and the changing dynamics of medical practice. I was not content to practice medicine with a factory floor mentality just to make a buck. My primary mantra in my medical practice is to always treat every patient of mine as a sister, and I could not in good conscience treat patients as if they were objects in a production line.

I hope that women who read this book will be able to prevent some medical conditions from developing, thus eliminating the need for a visit to a doctor's office. Prevention really is better than a cure. However, even with our best efforts at prevention, in some cases it is necessary to see a doctor. I am confident that this book will help readers be able to better describe their symptoms and get value for their dollars by making the most of their visit to the doctor's office. They will also be able to ask pertinent questions. While a book of this size cannot reasonably be expected to provide all the information on what one needs to know about women, I believe it is a starting point. Websites listed throughout the book create an additional avenue for those who need more information.

The Internet and our expanding access to it from homes, libraries, cafes, and offices allow anyone with the desire to learn limitless sources of all kinds of information. I have provided links to a variety of sites that provide medical and health information. Many more abound, and if this book provides the motivation for your initial foray of the Internet, it will have served one of its purposes.

We owe it to ourselves to become knowledgeable about our bodies and health. A better understanding of our bodies and the effects of various activities and choices will arm us with the necessary tools to make the changes that are important to ensuring our well-being. The Igbo people have a saying: "You lay on the mat that you make." As we mature, the early choices we make with respect to our life, our health, and our bodies are the things that determine the quality of our lives.

I have spiced this book with quotes and witty remarks—mostly by women—because I believe that in them lie wisdom and truisms from which we can all learn. If we choose not to do so, the Igbo have a another proverb, "the buttocks that are bitten by an ant soon learns where not to sit down." From that point of view, this book is aimed at preventing women from having to live it to learn it, from having to experience it to know it. Specifically, this book is primarily about preventive health and comprehensive education, and it will be deemed to be successful if one person finds it useful.

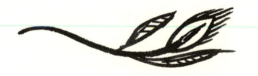

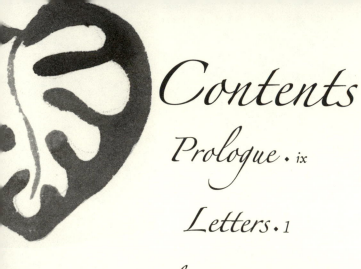

Contents

Prologue • ix

Letters • 1

Common Gynecologic Conditions • 109

Sexually Transmitted Diseases • 115

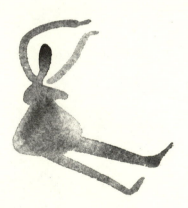

A woman's health is her capital.

HARRIET BEECHER STOWE

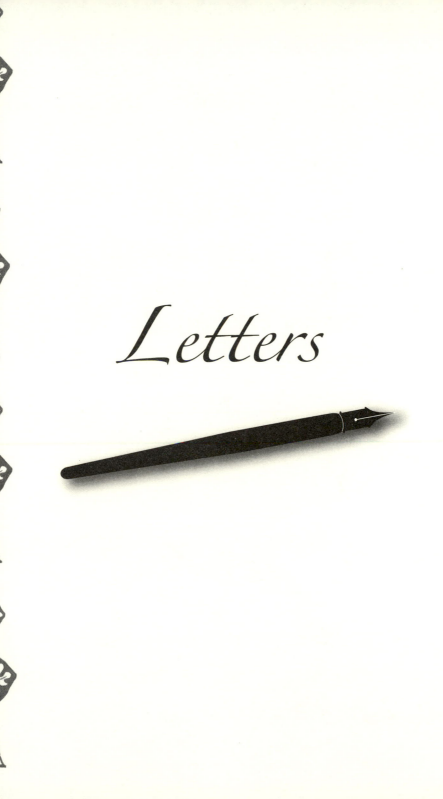

Letters

Asking questions is one of the fundamental keys of learning. It is always better to ask a question than pretend you understand.

CATHERINE PULSIFER

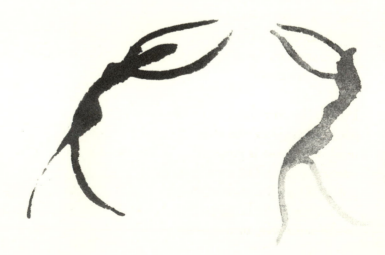

Dear Carolyn,

I am sorry I expressed surprise at your lack of knowledge of the female genitals. But you are so sophisticated in many ways, that even though I know of women who do not have a good understanding of their bodies I never imagined you to be one. I am even ashamed to admit that, until I graduated from High School, I thought my menstrual period and urine came from one hole.

After all, who should be the one teaching you about your body? My daughters are knowledgeable because their mother is a physician, but for those who do not have relatives with the requisite knowledge, where should they get their information? Talking about my daughters, I will relate this story: In school, while learning letters of the alphabet and the words that can be formed with them, the teacher came to the letter P and asked my daughter what words started with the letter. My daughter, in all her innocence, said "penis." I was not in the classroom, but the teacher's tone when she called me to relate the story showed that she must have been alarmed by my daughter's answer. What does a mother do in such a situation? I told her not to worry, that in our household, we were very forthcoming about using the right words every time.

I think the best thing to do is to get a mirror and one of those book lights. Don't be afraid to look at your body. What you immediately see is your vulva. You have hair on the sides that extend upward. The area that has the most hair is called the mons pubis. When you look at the sides, the area that most lay people call the lip is the labia majora. For some women, both sides might be the same size, or one side may be bigger than the other. When you separate the labia majora, you will see the labia minora. It is so important to clean between the labia majora and labia minora on both sides. If discharge gets in this area, it becomes irritated. If you follow the labia minora upward, it splits and forms a hood on top. This is the area of the clitoris. Below the clitoris, you will notice a hole. This is the urethra, where urine comes out. Below this hole is another one, the introitus, which is the entryway to the vagina.

It is important when wiping after urination to wipe from front to back. Wiping from the back, where there are more bacteria, to the front could create problems, including bacterial vaginosis.

Again, I apologize for the way I expressed my amazement during your visit. I applaud you for asking the question. I have enclosed three detailed drawings that you should find helpful. One shows the external genitalia I have described here. The second and third drawings will help you understand the internal anatomy of the female reproductive organs. If you have any more questions, please feel free to schedule an appointment.

Sincerely,

Ngozi Osuagwu, MD, FACOG

External Genitalia

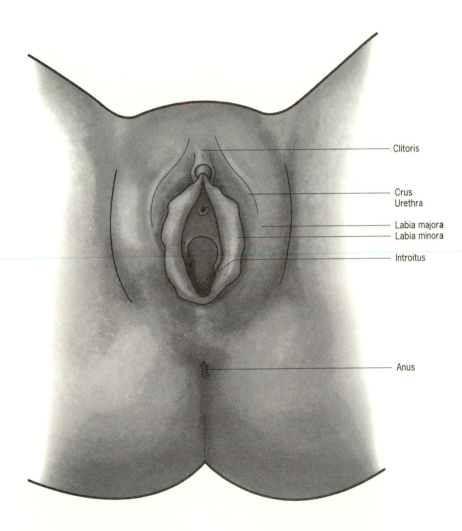

Clitoris

Crus
Urethra

Labia majora
Labia minora

Introitus

Anus

Ovary, Fallopian Tube, Uterus and Vagina

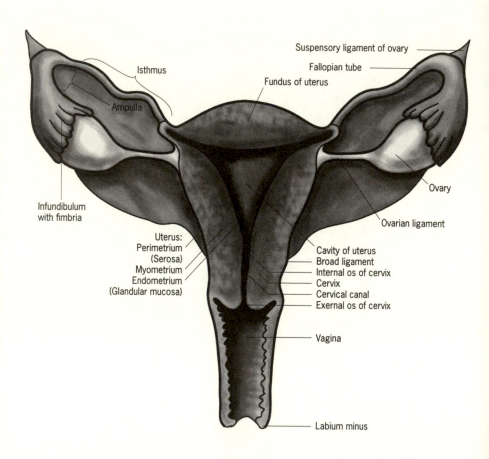

Suspensory ligament of ovary

Fallopian tube

Fundus of uterus

Isthmus

Ampulla

Ovary

Infundibulum
with fimbria

Ovarian ligament

Uterus:
Perimetrium
(Serosa)
Myometrium
Endometrium
(Glandular mucosa)

Cavity of uterus
Broad ligament
Internal os of cervix
Cervix
Cervical canal
Exernal os of cervix

Vagina

Labium minus

Female Pelvic Organs

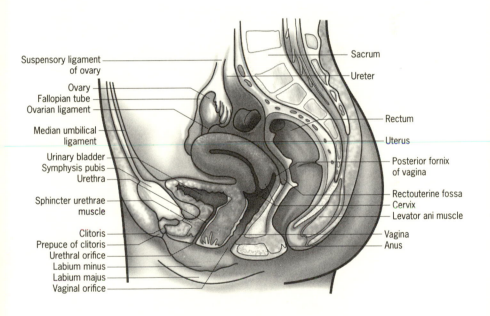

Suspensory ligament of ovary

Ovary

Fallopian tube

Ovarian ligament

Median umbilical ligament

Urinary bladder

Symphysis pubis

Urethra

Sphincter urethrae muscle

Clitoris

Prepuce of clitoris

Urethral orifice

Labium minus

Labium majus

Vaginal orifice

Sacrum

Ureter

Rectum

Uterus

Posterior fornix of vagina

Rectouterine fossa

Cervix

Levator ani muscle

Vagina

Anus

... it is the greatest of all mistakes to begin life with the expectation that it is going to be easy, or with the wish to have it so.

 LUCY LARCOM

Dear Abigail,

You called to ask about what tests you are required to have as part of your prenatal care. There are several tests that your physician will order during your prenatal visits. The tests that the physician orders depend on how far along you are in pregnancy and any risk factors you might have based on your medical and family history.

Most pregnant women come to their physician during the first trimester. The doctor will give you a physical exam. During this exam, a pap smear and cultures for gonorrhea and chlamydia will be obtained. The Pap smear is a screening test for cervical cancer. If this test is abnormal, you will need further testing. If the gonorrhea or chlamydia results are positive, you and your partner will need to be treated with antibiotics and then retested to confirm that the infection has been eliminated.

Your physician will also order several blood tests. The complete blood count (CBC) is a test to screen for anemia. Your blood will also be typed, and it will be screened for antibodies. Your blood will be screened for syphilis and hepatitis as well. A rubella test will be ordered, and lack of immunity will require you to be vaccinated after delivering the baby. HIV testing will also be offered, but your blood will be tested only with your permission. Knowledge of your status assists the doctor in determining the method of managing your care to decrease the chances of transmission to the child. A urine test to check for infection is also ordered.

Depending on your risk factors, you might be screened for cystic fibrosis and sickle cell disease. Other tests might be ordered depending on your ancestry. If you are of Eastern European or

Ashkenazi Jewish ancestry, it may be important to test for Tay-Sach's disease. These screening tests are mostly elective and will only be done if you agree to have them done.

Between fifteen and nineteen weeks of pregnancy, you will be asked if you want to be screened for neural tube defects (problems with the spine of the baby) and Down's syndrome. If you want to be screened, you will have an alpha fetal protein test. This test may be enhanced with further tests to make the screening more valuable. Between twenty-four and twenty-eight weeks, you will be screened for diabetes with a one-hour glucose challenge test. Depending on the result of the test, you may have to do the three-hour glucose tolerance test to determine if you have gestational diabetes. This is diabetes that is diagnosed during pregnancy but usually resolves after pregnancy. Between thirty-five and thirty-seven weeks of pregnancy, you will be screened for group B streptococcus infection. Cultures will be obtained from your vagina and rectum. If this test is positive, you will need antibiotics when you go into labor.

I cannot overemphasize the importance of early prenatal care. Am I correct in assuming that you are not making an appointment has to do with insurance coverage? Is it that you do not have any insurance coverage at this time and you are waiting to be covered by your job? Are you concerned that your insurance will not cover you for the pregnancy because it will be deemed to be a pre-existing condition, and so not liable for coverage? The only advice I can give is that you start taking vitamins immediately and make an appointment as early as you can.

Sincerely,

Ngozi Osuagwu, MD, FACOG

The One in the Glass

When you get what you want in your struggle for self,
And the world dubs you queen, or king for a day
Just go to a mirror and look at yourself,
And see what it has to say.

For it isn't your mother, father, husband, or wife,
Whose judgment upon you must pass.
The one whose verdict counts most in your life,
Is the one staring back from the glass.

Some people might think you're an honorable chum,
And call you a great gal, or guy.
But one in the glass says you're only a bum,
If you can't look yourself straight in the eye.

You're the one to please, never mind all the rest,
For it's you alone, clear up to the end.
And you've passed your most dangerous, difficult test,
If the one in the glass is your friend.

You may fool the masses down the pathway of years,
And get pats on the back, as you pass.
But your final reward will be heartache and tears,
If you've cheated the one in the glass.

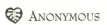 ANONYMOUS

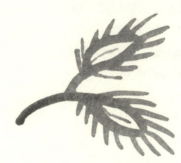

An ounce of prevention is worth a
pound of cure.

 PROVERB

Dear Karen,

I am writing to repeat what I said yesterday. Although everything I said was correct, upon further contemplation, I may not have communicated in my best bedside manner. I apologize for the manner in which I reacted to you during the visit. However, my apology should not be inferred as a change of my view that you are not a candidate for gastric bypass surgery.

During your visit, you wanted me to clear you for gastric bypass surgery. And as you remember, I asked you for the results of the psychological profile given to candidates for this procedure. You said you passed, but there appears to be a problem. You told me that you did not have any time to exercise, and you failed to respond fully to my questions about your dietary habits.

How, then, can I in good conscience clear you for such a surgery? I feel that if you were as honest in completing the profile as you were with me during our discussions, you would not have been cleared for the gastric bypass surgery. Based on our conversation, you are not yet ready for the procedure.

But we can do one of two things. We can begin developing the habits necessary for a successful long-term outcome, or you can choose to find another physician to clear you for the surgery. If you choose to look for another physician, I am sure you will find one eventually who will clear you for the surgery. If, however, you choose to start exercising, you can join our small exercise club, or any other club for that matter. If you start, we will watch your progress with exercising and re-evaluate your readiness for the surgery in another couple of months or so. If you choose to join The Healthy Woman, we will gladly waive some of the fees.

Let me restate what I expect you know already. The gastric bypass surgery reduces the size of your stomach, which means that you cannot eat as much after the procedure is performed. Changing your relationship with food by altering your dietary habits assures us that you will not overload the smaller stomach after the surgery. Exercising regularly improves your metabolism and ensures that you are able to get the most nutrients and energy from your decreased food intake after the procedure.

I hope this letter communicates how much I want to help. I also hope I have been open and honest in our communication. Keep me informed about what you choose to do. And of course, I am glad that you trust me enough to be your gynecologist as well as your primary care physician.

Sincerely,

Ngozi Osuagwu, MD, FACOG

Just as women's bodies are softer than men's, so their understanding is sharper.

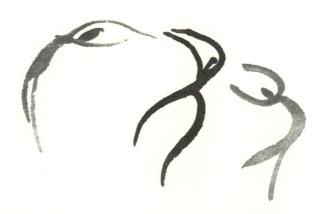 CHRISTINE DE PISAN

Dear Tonisha,

Recently we discussed management options for your uterine fibroids. You informed me that you have been experiencing heavy menstrual periods for the past eighteen months and you were beginning to experience lightheadedness with each period. You also told me that I am the fourth doctor you have seen in the past eighteen months.

Your medical history shows that you are thirty-eight years old and the mother of four children, the last of which you had about ten years ago. Your history also shows that the fibroids have grown steadily in the past five years, from the size of a grapefruit to the size of a cantaloupe. With your blood count so low, it borders on a miracle that you are still walking around. What I am saying is that you have lost a lot of blood, which has caused the hemoglobin level in your blood to drop below normal. The level has become too low to effectively transport oxygen to help the breakdown of food and the creation of energy, which explains why you are always tired.

I know you came to me because you heard that I am conservative in the management of uterine fibroids. It was also clear from our conversation that you hoped I would validate your opinion that you should keep your uterus. In most cases, that is exactly what I inform my patients. But each case is different, and in your case, having a hysterectomy (removing your uterus) is quite reasonable.

You are probably going to talk to some of your friends, who may ask whether you are getting a partial or complete hysterectomy. What they are asking is whether or not the ovaries will be removed along with the uterus. In some cases, when we remove the uterus, we also remove the ovaries. The procedure to remove the ovaries is known as an oophorectomy.

When talking about hysterectomies, we can also talk about having a total versus a subtotal hysterectomy. The difference involves your cervix—the mouth of the uterus. If the cervix is taken out, the procedure is a total hysterectomy. If the cervix is left in, the procedure is a subtotal or supracervical hysterectomy. Some people feel that leaving the cervix benefits you sexually; others disagree. The cervix can also support the vagina. We can discuss this in more detail during your next visit.

You may also be interested in knowing how I will remove your uterus. In a hysterectomy, the uterus can be removed through the vagina or the abdomen. When we do the surgery through the abdomen, it can be done with a large incision or with smaller incisions using the laparoscope. This is called a total abdominal hysterectomy (or TAH). When the removal is done through the vagina, it is called a total vaginal hysterectomy (or TVH), or when we use a laparoscope through the abdomen and remove the uterus through the vagina, it is called a laparoscopically assisted vaginal hysterectomy (LAVH). The method of surgery is determined based on the size of your uterus. The size of your uterus is too large for the minimally invasive procedure using a laparoscope, so we need to do the total abdominal hysterectomy.

Let me restate, after evaluating your case, you are not a candidate for the procedure that "Condoleeza Rice had to take care of her fibroids", which you mentioned during your visit. The procedure is called uterine artery embolization, and is performed by specialists called interventional radiologists. In this procedure, small plastic pellets are placed in the arteries that supply blood to the uterus. This stops the growth of the fibroids. As your obstetrician-gynecologist, I would refer you to an interventional radiologist if I felt it was the best option for you. To completely put you at ease, please call the office for us to schedule an appointment for you to see an interventional radiologist for a second opinion. I believe getting a second opinion is always a good idea.

After seeing the interventional radiologist and during your next visit to my office when we discuss the hysterectomy surgery in greater detail, we will also need to make a determination on whether you want your ovaries removed at the same time. The average age of menopause is fifty one. You are only thirty eight years old and have at least thirteen years of ovarian function left. Although there are risks of ovarian cancer, which is similar to every woman who has ovaries, I believe that the benefits of keeping your ovaries outweigh those risks, especially because you have no family history of ovarian cancer.

Our major goal now is to work on getting your blood count up while you consider your options. Because your hemoglobin level is too low, we have to build it up before we can perform the surgery. To increase your hemoglobin level, we will try to get you to bleed less and increase the level of iron in your blood. If we are not able to raise your hemoglobin to the required level before surgery, the only option we have may be to consider blood transfusion. Please call the office at your earliest convenience to schedule an appointment.

Sincerely,

Ngozi Osuagwu, MD, FACOG

Think before you act.

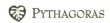 Pythagoras

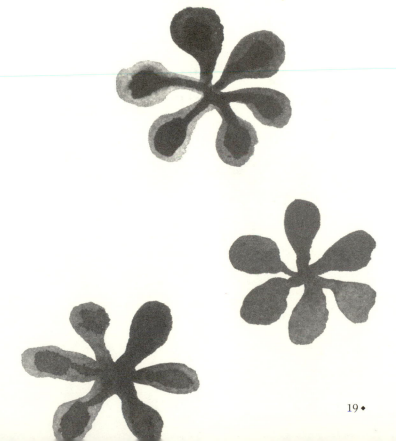

Self control isn't everything; it's
just that there's nothing without it.

GLORIA STEINEM

Dear Karla,

My God, couldn't you have thought of other things to do when you were upset with your husband? I believe that was the question I asked you during your visit the other day. I believe I may have acted in a self-righteous manner.

When you came in to see me and had a positive pregnancy test, I assumed that your husband was going to be a daddy again. And then you told me it was an old friend. I was stunned. When you started crying and asked to be left alone for a while, I obliged and left the room to see another patient, but I returned to find that you were gone.

I apologize for my reaction, and am sorry if you considered it judgmental. Who am I to judge your behavior? I should have controlled my response, but like everyone else, doctors are capable of being surprised and making mistakes. At this point in my career, I am at a stage where nothing surprises or shocks me, but surprise you did surprise me. If it makes it any better, my response would have been the same if my sister told me a story like that. Once more, please accept my sincere apology.

Because we never got a chance to discuss your options, I'll try to lay them out in this letter. These are various options I am sure you may have already considered. One option is to tell your husband. While we cannot predict his reaction, he may opt to stay in the marriage and support you with the pregnancy and raising the baby. You may also choose not to reveal to him the manner in which you got pregnant, and I am sure you will not be the first person to withhold such information. Leaving your husband and keeping the baby is another alternative worthy of consideration. Yet another option is to even consider terminating the pregnancy. And finally, you may also wish to give the baby up for adoption. In any choice you make, you have to be guided by your conscience.

Unfortunately, I can't make this decision for you. But whatever your choice, I'll support you. I am here for you.

Sincerely,

Ngozi Osuagwu, MD, FACOG

Less than one percent of the
people in the world reach their
full potential—and the
reason is they take their focus
off what they were doing.

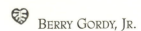 BERRY GORDY, JR.

Dear Asia,

I understand you are no longer with your baby's daddy. Look at me lapsing into calling your child's father "baby's daddy"—I like the ring of this new phrase. I never got to know him, but when I ran into your mother the other day she said he's currently with someone else. His lack of attention to you may explain why we did not connect.

So I think it's time that you begin to think about yourself. Remember, when you first came to see me, you were in high school with dreams of becoming a nurse. You finished high school two years ago. You now have a baby who will be two years old soon. The baby should not be an impediment and I believe you can still be a nurse. Yes, it will be more difficult, but you can still do it.

There are many avenues available for you to continue your education. My advice is to befriend a librarian who can help you find the programs and grant opportunities available to young single mothers like yourself. There are many libraries around your neighborhood and nothing makes most of the librarians in the metropolitan library system happier than helping enthusiastic readers and researchers. I believe your mother will help if she knows that you have decided to make something of yourself. My hospital, like many others, has a tuition reimbursement program that is offered to employees working towards a professional health-oriented degree. You can contact the Human Resources offices at the hospital where I delivered your baby and mention that I suggested you explore available opportunities.

You also told me that this baby was an accident. Let us strive to prevent future accidents. You need to consider birth control.

There are many contraceptive options—the pill, the shot, the patch, and the ring to name a few. They can be used along with condoms. Why the condom? Because the condom may reduce the likelihood of contracting a sexually transmitted infection like the one you had during your pregnancy. Why have I not included abstinence? You know, it is the best method of contraception, and your guess is as good as mine on why I almost forgot to include it as an option. You need to get your life together and quickly because you are now a mother with responsibilities to a child.

A comprehensive discussion of contraception is too much to discuss in this letter. Please find enclosed with this letter a brochure, which reviews the different forms of contraception. If you would like to have a detailed discussion of this topic, please call the office and schedule an appointment.

Sincerely,

Ngozi Osuagwu MD, FACOG

Depression is nourished
by a lifetime of ungrieved
and unforgiven hurts.

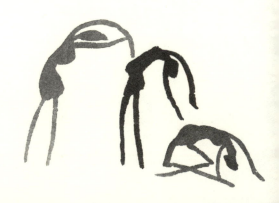 PENELOPE SWEET

Dear Elaine,

I am glad to see that you are doing so well on the new antidepressant medication that I prescribed. However, I want to emphasize that you still need counseling. It is important to state clearly that I am not going to prescribe any more medicines for you until you see a psychologist or a psychiatrist. In all honesty, they are the specialists who are experts that can deal with your concerns. As I tell my husband, who occasionally wants me to treat him, I am a specialist for women in the areas between their knees and belly buttons. My training allows me to recognize depression, treat it on a short term or emergency basis, and then refer you to the appropriate mental health provider. There may be a new medication that is available of which I am not aware, and or a novel technique available to help you. The experts will have that information.

Depression affects individuals completely. It affects you physically, emotionally, and mentally, and influences your sleep and eating habits, the way you feel about yourself and your thought process. Depression is not to be mistaken with the passing dour or blue mood. It is important to get the correct treatment, without which the symptoms can persist for a very long time. The symptoms vary depending on the individual and the intensity is related to the severity of the disease. There are different forms of depression and only the specialist can recognize and develop a plan for properly managing your care.

I know that you are afraid to seek counseling because of the stigma associated with mental illness. I know you do not want anybody to know. Let me be absolutely clear, depression is not a sign of personal weakness. Did you know that depression affects women twice the rate it affects men, and this is true regardless of ethnicity, economic status or race?

I know you are a beautiful person—one that needs help. I will be with you, but you need specialized care beyond the scope of my training and I will be doing you a disservice if I continue to manage your care with respect to depression. We will schedule an appointment with one of the specialists on the list I provided to you, once you give us the go ahead. Let us start the process of this healing immediately and make the appointment with the specialist.

Sincerely,

Ngozi Osuagwu, MD, FACOG

If you doubt you can accomplish something, then you can't accomplish it. You have to have the confidence in your ability, and then be tough enough to follow through.

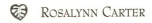 ROSALYNN CARTER

Dear Jaleen,

You are fat! How else do you expect me to put it? I could employ avoidance by sugar-coating things and saying that you are too short for your weight. But whom would I be fooling? You are 5'4", weighing 300 pounds, and have a body mass index of 51. By definition, you are grossly obese, and I would be doing you an injustice if I did not say so. Knowing what I know, it would be disingenuous for me not to be alarmed. I am writing because I care. I am not going to apologize for caring.

You need to make some life style changes and create a weight loss plan. In trying to lose and maintain a reasonable weight, there are no quick fixes—it is going to be a slow process requiring discipline, commitment, and diligence. I know that many fad diets offer quick results, but they do not represent a real solution. Fad diets often result in weight loss the first two weeks, but most people regain their weight and add more.

My advice is that you start slowly: A journey of a thousand miles starts with one step. And remember, it didn't take you one month to gain the weight, so it won't take you one month to lose it. I have read somewhere that slow and steady wins the race. First take a look at what you are eating. Does it have any nutritional value? Are these food items healthy? What can be eliminated? Spend time gradually eliminating these things. Try to stick with fresh and frozen food items and to keep in mind portion size.

Next, or as part of your diet, you have to become active. Exercise! Exercise! Exercise! Find an activity you enjoy and get moving. Do not tell me you do not have the time to exercise. We all find time for the things we consider important. I hope you are important to yourself. Remember that if you die tomorrow, the world keeps moving. Exercise is an investment in your future. With the ever-increasing cost of medication and medical care, and the reduction in insurance coverage, it pays to start habits that aid you in keeping healthy.

If I sound angry, it is because I am. I only want the best for you. How can I not be angry when down the hall from my office, in the nephrology office I see dialysis patients, among others? In most cases, the reason for kidney failure and the need for dialysis stems from obesity. Do me a favor and go online and study the effects of obesity. And please don't look at me and pretend that 5'4 and 300 lbs is okay. It is not okay and I won't lie about it. Please find attached to this letter a BMI chart for your review. Anyone with a BMI of greater than 25 is considered overweight.

I hope that your decision to switch health care providers marks the beginning of taking care of yourself. Good luck with your next doctor. I hope he or she will be just as concerned as I am.

Sincerely,

Ngozi Osuagwu MD, FACOG

BODY MASS INDEX TABLE FOR ADULTS

	NORMAL						OVERWEIGHT					OBESE						
BMI	19	20	21	22	23	24	25	26	27	28	29	30	31	32	33	34	35	36
Height (inches)	Body Weight (pounds)																	
58	91	96	100	105	110	115	119	124	129	134	138	143	148	153	158	162	167	172
59	94	99	104	109	114	119	124	128	133	138	143	148	153	158	163	168	173	178
60	97	102	107	112	118	123	128	133	138	143	148	153	158	163	168	174	179	184
61	100	106	111	116	122	127	132	137	143	148	153	158	164	169	174	180	185	190
62	104	109	115	120	126	131	136	142	147	153	158	164	169	175	180	186	191	196
63	107	113	118	124	130	135	141	146	152	158	163	169	175	180	186	191	197	203
64	110	116	122	128	134	140	145	151	157	163	169	174	180	186	192	197	204	209
65	114	120	126	132	138	144	150	156	162	168	174	180	186	192	198	204	210	216
66	118	124	130	136	142	148	155	161	167	173	179	186	192	198	204	210	216	223
67	121	127	134	140	146	153	159	166	172	178	185	191	198	204	211	217	223	230
68	125	131	138	144	151	158	164	171	177	184	190	197	203	210	216	223	230	236
69	128	135	142	149	155	162	169	176	182	189	196	203	209	216	223	230	236	243
70	132	139	146	153	160	167	174	181	188	195	202	209	216	222	229	236	243	250
71	136	143	150	157	165	172	179	186	193	200	208	215	222	229	236	243	250	257
72	140	147	154	162	169	177	184	191	199	206	213	221	228	235	242	250	258	265
73	144	151	159	166	174	182	189	197	204	212	219	227	235	242	250	257	265	272
74	148	155	163	171	179	186	194	202	210	218	225	233	241	249	256	264	272	280
75	152	160	168	176	184	192	200	208	216	224	232	240	248	256	264	272	279	287
76	156	164	172	180	189	197	205	213	221	230	238	246	254	263	271	279	287	295

The first step in managing obesity is to assess where you are. This can be done using your body mass index (BMI) and waist circumference. The BMI is based on a ratio of weight to height. If you know your weight in pounds and your height in inches, you can calculate your body mass index. Multiply your weight in pounds by 703 (A). Multiply your height (inches) and your height (in inches) (B). Divide A by B and you will get your BMI.

$$\frac{\text{Weight (pounds)} \times 703}{\text{Height (inches)} \times \text{Height (inches)}}$$

To get the BMI of a woman who is five feet nine inches and weighs one hundred and fifty pounds from the chart:
1. Find the woman height in inches. 69 inches.
2. We know her weight is 150 pounds.
3. Find the height on the first line and using your fingers, find the weight closest to 150 pounds. It is 149. Run your fingers straight up and you will see that she has a BMI of 22.

/I	37	38	39	40	41	42	43	44	45	46	47	48	49	50	51	52	53	54
ight ches)	Body Weight (pounds)																	
	177	181	186	191	196	201	205	210	215	220	224	229	234	239	244	248	253	258
	183	188	193	198	203	208	212	217	222	227	232	237	242	247	252	257	262	267
	189	194	199	204	209	215	220	225	230	235	240	245	250	255	261	266	271	276
	195	201	206	211	217	222	227	232	238	243	248	254	259	264	269	275	280	285
	202	207	213	218	224	229	235	240	246	251	256	262	267	273	278	284	289	295
	208	214	220	225	231	237	242	248	254	259	265	270	278	282	287	293	299	304
	215	221	227	232	238	244	250	256	262	267	273	279	285	291	296	302	308	314
	222	228	234	240	246	252	258	264	270	276	282	288	294	300	306	312	318	324
	229	235	241	247	253	260	266	272	278	284	291	297	303	309	315	322	328	334
	236	242	249	255	261	268	274	280	287	293	299	306	312	319	325	331	338	344
	243	249	256	262	269	276	282	289	295	302	308	315	322	328	335	341	348	354
	250	257	263	270	277	284	291	297	304	311	318	324	331	338	345	351	358	365
	257	264	271	278	285	292	299	306	313	320	327	334	341	348	355	362	369	376
	265	272	279	286	293	301	308	315	322	329	338	343	351	358	365	372	379	386
	272	279	287	294	302	309	316	324	331	338	346	353	361	368	375	383	390	397
	280	288	295	302	310	318	325	333	340	348	355	363	371	378	386	393	401	408
	287	295	303	311	319	326	334	342	350	358	365	373	381	389	396	404	412	420
	295	303	311	319	327	335	343	351	359	367	375	383	391	399	407	415	423	431
	304	312	320	328	336	344	353	361	369	377	385	394	402	410	418	426	435	443

Source: National Heart, Lung and Blood Institute Website. Adapted from Clinical Guidelines on the Identification, Evaluation, and Treatment of Overweight and Obesity in Adults:The Evidence Report.

If the number is less than 18.5, you are underweight. If it is between 18.5 and 24.9, you are normal weight, 25.0 to 29.9 is overweight. 30.0 to 39.9 is obese and greater that or equal to 40.0 is extreme obesity. This formula does not work well for the elderly or the muscular athlete. A waist circumference for men greater than 40 inches and for women greater than 35 inches puts one at risk for significant cardiovascular disease. If your BMI is greater than 35, don't bother checking waist circumference, you are at risk for the chronic diseases mentioned above.

There are two parts to losing weight or maintaining weight. You have to watch what goes in your body and on the other side of the equation you have to be prepared to exert energy. Studies have shown that people who have been successful with controlling their weight had four common behaviors: they ate a low calorie, low-fat diet, monitored their weight frequently, were very physically fit and ate breakfast.

Dear Shakira,

I did not perform a Pap smear during your last appointment. I simply performed a pelvic exam and took cultures. The cultures will enable us to better evaluate the medical condition that brought you to my office, and of course treat you properly.

You are not due for a Pap smear for another six months. People always seem to confuse a pelvic exam and a pap smear, but these terms are not synonymous. A Pap smear and an annual gynecological examination are also not the same. Another common misconception is that a Pap smear is done whenever a pelvic exam is conducted, but a Pap smear is only one of the tests that can be done during a pelvic exam.

During a pelvic exam, I examine the genitalia. Although I know you may have heard your genitalia referred to as a coochie, pocketbook, or another common slang term, the correct name is actually the vulva. I insert a speculum into the vagina to enable me to view inside the vagina, and check for bleeding, discharge, or any lesions. I also take a look at the cervix, which is the mouth of the uterus. I then perform a bimanual examination. This is where I insert two fingers into the vagina and place my other hand on the abdomen to feel for the other pelvic organs, which include the uterus and ovaries.

Other tests may include those to check for sexually transmitted infections like gonorrhea and chlamydia, or if you are bleeding abnormally, an endometrial biopsy. There are still other tests that I may conduct to check the uterus, fallopian tubes, and ovaries for normal development.

Pap smears are recommended for all women over twenty-one years of age, or earlier if they are sexually active. Some people, especially Spanish speakers, refer to the Pap test as Papinicolaou, after George Papinicolaou, who developed the test. Its main purpose is to screen for cervical cancer. A sample is collected by gently scraping the loose cells at the opening of the cervix. The collected cells are placed on slides or in a bottle and examined for any abnormalities. I must point out that the Pap smear only serves to screen for cervical cancer. It does not tell us anything about ovarian, breast or endometrial cancer. Please note that the best time for a Pap smear is before or after your menstrual period, and best results are obtained if you do not douche, use any medication in your vagina, or have sexual intercourse for twenty four hours before your Pap is done.

An annual exam is a head to toe examination. It includes examining the teeth, listening to the heart and lungs, and performing breast, abdominal, and pelvic exams. A Pap smear may be performed during an annual examination, but it is not required.

I hope you have a better knowledge of what we mean by pelvic examinations and pap smears. The next time you have a pelvic examination, you should feel free to ask why it is being done. Do not assume it is only to obtain a pap smear.

Sincerely,

Ngozi Osuagwu, MD, FACOG

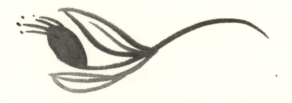

I wonder if one of the penalties of growing older is that you become more and more conscious that nothing in life is very permanent.

ELEANOR ROOSEVELT

Dear Josephine,

The last time you came in to the office to see me, I thought we would have to use a mop to wipe the floor! I had not realized that your hot flashes were so bad. I'm also sorry I had to rush out for a delivery in the middle of your appointment, although I believe we covered most of the risks and benefits of the use of hormone replacement therapy.

Now, how do we begin to address the problem that brought you in for the appointment? I have reviewed your chart and gathered enough information from your personal history and that of your family to offer a suggestion. All the same, the final decision is yours. Because your symptoms are so severe that it impacts your ability to function at your work place, I believe that you would benefit from hormone replacement therapy. Since you have a uterus (you have not had a hysterectomy), you will need to take both estrogen and progesterone. There are many delivery systems available. You can take the hormones orally (by mouth) or apply them on your skin through a patch. There are also creams and rings that contain hormones, but neither contains a combination of estrogen and progesterone.

There are many reports regarding both the benefits and risks of hormone replacement therapy (HRT). We know that HRT helps with hot flashes and that it helps decrease the risk of osteoporosis (weakening of bone mass). We also know that there are some risks from hormone replacement therapy. The more common risks include strokes, breast cancer, and clots in the deep veins (deep vein thrombosis). These clots, while not life threatening, are associated with potentially fatal conditions. A dislodged clot can cause difficulty breathing or can cause a stroke if it gets lodged in the lungs or the brain. My job as your physician is to assess each patient as an individual and make a determination on the pros and cons of prescribing hormones.

I would like you to come back to the office so I can review this information with you. I know it was my fault that the last office visit was not complete; you will not have to pay the co-payment on this next visit.

Sincerely,

Ngozi Osuagwu, MD FACOG

...men know best about everything,
except what women know better.

GEORGE ELIOT

Dear Rebecca,

I know you were upset that I didn't call in yet another prescription for "yeast infection," as you requested. As a doctor who strives for excellence, I cannot in good conscience prescribe any additional medication without seeing you. Not every discharge with itching is a yeast infection. More importantly, this was the third time in four months that you requested and I have called in a prescription for a "yeast infection." Obviously, something else may be wrong. So you do need to schedule an appointment for us to evaluate and diagnose whatever is happening.

There are many causes of discharge from the vagina. You could have a sexually transmitted disease such as gonorrhea or chlamydia, which means you should be tested. These are serious diseases and often present no symptoms, but they can cause problems later that may affect your reproductive ability. Have you ever wondered why so many young people are struggling to have children? Many are finding out that sexually transmitted diseases have wreaked havoc on their reproductive system, making it difficult to conceive. These diseases create scar tissue. The scar tissue can block the fallopian tubes, which are the conduits for the zygote (formed after fertilization of the egg by the sperm) as it migrates to implant in the uterus. In some cases, scarring caused by a sexually transmitted disease may cause ectopic pregnancies. This happens when the zygote starts to develop in the fallopian tubes rather than in the uterus. Failure to treat any sexually transmitted disease promptly can lead to chronic pain, which may not be helped by any medicine. They can also cause pelvic inflammatory disease (also known as PID).

Your infection may also be due to vaginitis. The most common causes of vaginitis are bacterial vaginosis, trichomoniasis, and yeast. Prescriptions to combat yeast infections won't help you with the first two. Bacterial vaginosis is usually associated with odor but not itching, while trichomoniasis is associated with both odor and itching. Both diseases need antibiotics for treatment. If we diagnose trichomoniasis, your partner also needs to be treated because trichomoniasis, unlike bacterial vaginosis, is sexually transmitted.

With all these possibilities, I can neither make a diagnosis over the telephone nor continue to call in prescriptions. Please make an appointment so that I can evaluate you fully and also obtain samples for a culture. I hope that after you have read this letter you understand why it is important for us to see you in the office. We hope to see you soon.

Sincerely,

Ngozi Osuagwu, MD, FACOG

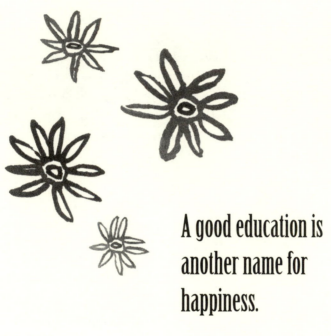

A good education is
another name for
happiness.

ANN PLATO

Dear Lansing,

Congratulations! Your mother gave me the good news that you have been accepted into The Johns Hopkins University, which was your first choice. She also told me this would be your first time away from home. I am proud of your accomplishments and I am flattered you chose to attend my alma mater. I am also very proud of you for choosing to attend an out of state college. Buckeyes are notorious for attending school from kindergarten through graduate school in Ohio, so it is refreshing to find that you chose to attend school outside of Ohio.

As I reminisce, I remember seeing you two years ago when you had problems with your menstrual cycle. I'm glad that the pain has decreased with the high dose of Ibuprofen I prescribed. As you may recall, I did not perform a pelvic exam at that time because you were not sexually active. You have a good head on your shoulders, and I know you understand that should you choose to become sexually active, you need to see a gynecologist first and have a comprehensive conversation about the topic.

A lot will happen while you are away. While at college you may find that special person that you want to date. Dating the right person can actually be beneficial to your college experience, and I want to state clearly that dating should not necessarily include sex. Let me be clear; I would really prefer that you wait until marriage to engage in sexual intercourse. Am I being a prude? If you know me, you know I am blunt with these matters. I realize, however, that I am living in the real world and my preference may be somewhat idealistic. Either way, you need to understand everything about sex, contraception, and sexually transmitted infections before you become sexually active.

There are lots of things for you to consider, but the two most important questions are: Am I ready? Is this the guy I want to be my first? You should never succumb to anyone until you are ready. Mind you, there will be pressure from both the young men and your girlfriends. However, always remember that it is your decision and yours alone.

I like to think of my body as a temple. Whatever I put in this temple has to be clean and worthy. When I talk about what you put in your temple, it includes food. Have you heard of the freshman 20? It refers to the 20 pounds many college freshmen gain as a result of all the junk food they eat. It is important to eat balanced meals that contain fruits, vegetables, nuts (if you are not allergic to them), grains, and some multivitamins to supplement what you get from your food.

Please do get some sleep. The temptation to party because no one is looking over your shoulders for the first time means you may not get enough sleep. Sleeping allows you to rejuvenate yourself. Remember that you are in college to study and not to party! Having said that, it is also important to let the college pass through you and not just pass through the college. Occasionally going to a jazz club or enjoying a meal in a nice seafood restaurant should not negatively impact your work. All I am saying is that we have to do everything in moderation.

Also, it is easier to make good grades and create a favorable impression on your professors in the first year. Demonstrating diligence, dedication, and ability to work hard will make the professors future advocates for you. Remember! First impression is the best impression. Developing and maintaining a good relationship with peers, professors, and all the staff at the school provides you with some support away from your family. Note that I mentioned the importance of also having a good relationship with the staff. You may not deal with them on a daily basis, but it is important that you recognize that good relationships with them can positively affect your stay in the school. You may also want to surround yourself with other positive people from your school's community and your place of worship.

I wish you well in your future endeavors. If you can, do stop by the office and say hello. If you can't visit before you go to school, good luck, and best wishes. Please do not hesitate to call if you have any questions.

Sincerely,

Ngozi Osuagwu, MD, FACOG

Of course, it is easy to turn your eyes from what is happening if it is not happening to you. Or if you have not put yourself where it is happening.

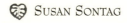 SUSAN SONTAG

Dear Rickie,

You tell me James feels disrespected because I do not communicate with him during your prenatal visits. Now that you raise the issue, have you ever stopped to consider how uncomfortable I feel in his presence, knowing that he may not be the father of your baby?

Well, I find it very difficult to look at such a devoted and doting companion who attends to your every need, never doubting he is your baby's father. I am tongue-tied. And you will have to come up with a way of telling him that my actions do not have anything to do with him. Telling him I am a very quiet doctor is an inconsequential fib compared to the lie we are living now. However, he may find it difficult to believe since I am sure he has overheard my roaring laughter from the other rooms during your prenatal visits.

I don't even know why I'm writing you. Maybe it's because I feel so guilty and I'm trying very hard not to view myself as an accomplice. Or maybe it's because I believe that as adults we must deal with the consequences of our actions. I will try my best to talk with him during your visits although I now have renewed respect for those Catholic priests who hear confessions.

You will be having this baby in two weeks. Shouldn't you let him know? After all, James has been extremely supportive of you. I am concerned. Suppose something happens and your baby needs a blood donor? Is that the best way for him to find out? I don't have the answer. You say if he finds out, he will "kill you." Well, then the other option is that we pray. We pray that the dates are correct and that James is the father.

I guess I just wanted you to know that I don't agree how you are handling this issue with respect to the determination of the child's paternity, but I will stand by you. You are my patient and your welfare is my first priority.

Sincerely,

Ngozi Osuagwu, MD, FACOG

I am still determined to be cheerful and happy in whatever situation I may be, for I have learned from experience that the greater part of our happiness or misery depends on our dispositions and not on our circumstances.

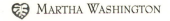 MARTHA WASHINGTON

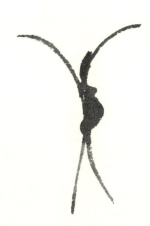

Dear Paula,

I have thought about it for some time, but I have decided that I cannot tie your tubes. You have only one child—albeit from an unexpected pregnancy—but I cannot in good conscience tie your tubes. My refusal is based on experience. And while I cannot mention names, it may be prudent to tell you this story.

Josephine, who was in her mid-thirties, decided after having two children that she was done with making babies. She wanted and requested permanent sterilization because she was also tired of taking birth control pills. She said she had not found the right man and she seldom engaged in sex when the opportunity arose. She had a frank and comprehensive discussion with her gynecologist and convinced him, because she had one child of each gender and was nearing what was considered at the time to be advanced maternal age (thirty five and above). Josephine had a bilateral tubal ligation.

Much to her gynecologist's chagrin, four years later she showed up with a sheepish grin asking for a tubal ligation reversal. Her knight in shining armor had just come charging in and she wanted to make a baby with him. The good news is that Josephine did have that baby, but the somewhat sad news is that it came at a huge expense, financially and emotionally.

So for you, my dear, Mr. Right may walk through the door tomorrow and both of you may decide to have another baby. I know my job is not to tell you what to do and that you will make the final decision. I am simply informing you of your options. This is an invasive procedure that is not always reversible.

It won't surprise me if you find some other doctor willing to do the procedure—after all, you are paying for it—but I won't be the one to do it. I know you don't want to take the pill because you are concerned about weight gain, but have you considered other methods of birth control? What do you think about an intrauterine device (IUD)? This is a good option if you are in a monogamous relationship and may want to have children later on. The intrauterine device looks like a T and is placed in the uterus. There are two types of IUDs, one that lasts for five years and the other that lasts for ten years. Also available for your consideration is the shot (Depo Provera®) that lasts for three months. Depo Provera® is given once every twelve weeks by an injection either to your arm or on your buttocks. Condoms and spermicides are other options. You are probably aware that condoms are sheaths that cover the penis and prevent sperm from being introduced into the reproductive tract. Spermicides are chemical products that are inserted into the vagina prior to sexual activity and act to kill or deactivate sperm. I can also fit you with a diaphragm. The diaphragm covers the cervix and prevents the entry of the sperm into the uterus. I urge you to seriously consider these other options before deciding to go through with the tubal ligation for permanent sterilization.

If you still want your tubes tied, I suggest you ask your friends to refer you to other possible gynecologists. You can also call the local medical association or use the yellow pages. If you want us to further discuss the other options that I outlined above, please call the office and schedule an appointment.

Sincerely,

Ngozi Osuagwu, MD, FACOG

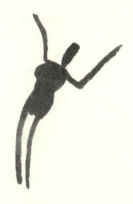

Laughter is one of the strongest
medicines on the planet … If it's strong
enough to kill an orgasm, surely it's
strong enough to kill cancer.

LOTUS WEINSTOCK

Dear Jesse,

I just received the report with your results. I have tried calling you several times but was unable to leave a message because there was no answering machine. I know you do not have any family here, so I want you to know that not only am I your physician, I am also your friend.

I spoke to the surgeon and was told that the biopsy confirmed breast cancer, but this is not a death sentence. You did everything right. You noticed a lump in your breast, immediately scheduled an appointment with me, and a mammogram and breast ultrasound was performed. Although the mammogram was normal and the breast ultrasound was questionable, you agreed to see the breast specialist because we both felt the lump. I am happy that we both took the lump seriously and did not ignore it.

So, what do we do now? We move on and tackle this problem head on. We cannot go back and pretend as if nothing has happened. The best thing we can do is to educate ourselves so that we understand all the options available. There are so many breast cancer survivors and I see us remembering this moment years from now and laughing at the scare like it was one of those phantom monsters from our childhood. Every day new medications are developed and we learn a little more about the management of this disease.

Do you know that women fear breast cancer almost twice as much as a heart attack even though each year the number of women who die of cardiovascular disease is twelve times as many women who die of breast cancer? Do you know that the number of people who die of breast cancer has progressively decreased beginning in the early 1990s? Did you know that more women die of lung cancer than breast cancer? While it is understandable that you are upset about the diagnosis, I tell you discovering it as early as we did makes your prognosis very promising.

I was reading in my book, *God's Little Daily Devotional*, "When I come to the end of my rope, God is there to take over." Please do not hide from me, or any of the people who have been trying to contact you. I am here for you as are all the extended family of your church. Allow us to share your burden and show we care for you.

Sincerely,

Ngozi Osuagwu, MD, FACOG

You don't get to choose how
you're going to die. Or when.
You can only decide how you're
going to live. Now.

 JOAN BAEZ

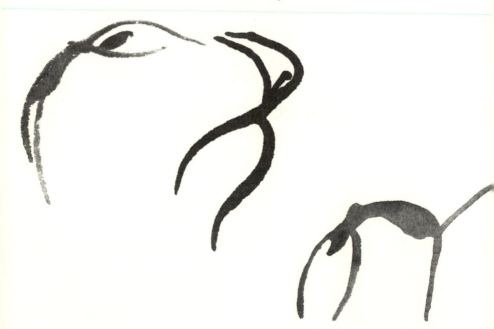

The key to the prison of
depression is simply to
become truly your own
best friend.

DOROTHY ROWE

Dear Nancy,

You ran out of my office so quickly after I gave you the diagnosis that I had no time to talk to you. I know you were upset about the diagnosis. It is true; you have herpes. It was confirmed by both the results of the culture I performed and the blood test I requested when you came for your last appointment.

Many women think that once they are over fifty and menopausal, they have nothing to worry about. And although you do not have to worry about getting pregnant, there are still sexually transmitted infections to which you can be exposed.

The good news is that herpes is not fatal. But it is a virus, which means there is no cure. There are two approaches we can take in the management of your disease. I can treat you for recurrent outbreaks, which will help shorten the amount of time you have symptoms. The other option is suppressive therapy. I usually reserve this approach for people who have frequent outbreaks (more than four times in a year), or patients with partners known not to have herpes. This therapy will help decrease the risk of transmitting the virus since most transmissions occur when the patient is asymptomatic, or without symptoms.

I am ready to work with you. Please schedule an appointment as soon as possible.

Sincerely,

Ngozi Osuagwu, MD, FACOG

An inquiring, analytical mind; an unquenchable thirst for new knowledge; and a heartfelt compassion for the ailing — these are prominent traits among the committed clinicians who have preserved the passion for medicine.

LOIS DeBAKEY

Dear Melissa,

I am not going to perform another myomectomy. I have already performed the procedure twice and I now have to recommend a hysterectomy. I recognize that because you do not have any children, you want to preserve your ability to have them one day. But Melissa, your fibroids have become enlarged again and your uterus is now the same size as that of a woman who is five months pregnant, and you are very anemic (your blood count is very low).

I wish I had something else to offer you, but I do not. I only suggest this surgery as a last resort, but if you are uneasy about it, you are well within your rights to get a second opinion. Never feel pressured to have any medical procedure. You must feel confident in your physician and their reasoning for performing a procedure.

At the rate this tumor is growing, it is obvious things are not looking good. You must also realize that a hysterectomy is not an easy solution. So while I want to make it clear that you need the procedure, I also want to make sure you understand the potential complications, which includes bleeding, infection, and possible injury to any nearby organ, particularly the bladder and/or bowel. Also, with each myomectomy, scar tissue forms around uterus, so it is difficult to gauge how much scar tissue you have prior to the surgery. The fortunate thing is that I performed the last surgery and you had minimal adhesions or scar tissue at that time. Believe me, I am not trying to scare you, but there are potential complications associated with almost every surgical procedure. I don't anticipate any of the complications mentioned, but they can happen.

I know your main concern has been maintaining your childbearing capacity. Once the hysterectomy is performed, you won't be able to have children in the traditional way. Since your ovaries will be left in, you might consider surrogacy. This is where your eggs are harvested from your ovaries and fertilized with your partner's sperm for a surrogate mother to carry. You also have the option of adoption.

By leaving your ovaries in, you will continue to experience all the emotional swings, bloating, and other symptoms associated with menstruation. The only thing you will not have is bleeding. This is because your uterus will be gone. If you have any questions, feel free to contact me at your convenience.

Sincerely,

Ngozi Osuagwu, MD, FACOG

To remove ignorance is
an important branch of
benevolence.

 ANN PLATO

Dear Petrie,

I am sorry, but I cannot help an eighteen-year old unemployed high school dropout get pregnant. For God's sake, you are just eighteen! Don't you want something better for your life? Don't you want something better for your child? I know that all your friends have babies, but that doesn't mean you must have one also. Babies are not the latest Coach or Prada handbags!

You should focus on trying to better yourself. A welfare check each month is not the same as a paycheck. Yes, you are right in saying that many people have done it, but I have never heard any of them say it was easy. Think about it; if you have a child now, what kind of future will you have? What of the baby? You'll be yet another single unemployed young mother struggling to raise a baby. I am sorry, but I won't be a part of it. I won't turn you into a statistic. As I have always believed, it is better to be poor alone than with a child.

Think about going back to school. Think about what you want for your future and how you can best help yourself and contribute to the society. Reflect on who you are. Why are you in this world? Is it only to have a baby? What can you add to this world? Go stand in front of a mirror and look at yourself. Introduce yourself to the person in the mirror. Do you like that person? Can that person be better than what you see now? I look at you and I say yes. Can it happen with a child straddled on your side? I say no.

Get a life! The longer I ponder your request, the more upset I get. Please do not come to my office with such requests. Please think about what I have said and do give me a call if you are ready to consider other ideas than having a baby. Actually, I want you to call the office and schedule an appointment with my secretary for me to treat you to lunch as soon as possible.

Sincerely,

Ngozi Osuagwu, MD, FACOG

We are each responsible for
our own life—no other
person is or even can be.

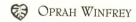 OPRAH WINFREY

Dear Bridget,

How can I help you? Your mother loves you so much and has done her best to raise you. You have grown up right in front of my eyes. I have seen you through gonorrhea and herpes. I have tried to protect you from getting pregnant. You tried pills, the shot, and then the patch. I have watched you join the growing population of high school dropouts. And now you will be an uneducated teenage mother.

I feel like shaking some sense into you. Granted the father of your baby is not the guy who gave you all those diseases, but you have only known him for four months. Like you, he is a high school dropout. What kind of future do you expect this child to have? How do I reach you? I wrote this letter because talking has not worked.

I hope that when you get this letter you realize that I truly care for you and your baby. I will take care of you the best way I can. I want the best for you, but I also realize you have got to want the best for your child. I am not talking about the latest Air Jordan sneakers or that fly outfit that he or she must be seen in. I am talking about creating a life of independence for you and your child and by you raising an educated individual who can make reasonable decisions. I am talking about raising a self-confident individual, an individual who knows how to use all the resources available to him or her.

Bridget, do something with your life. I suggest you start studying for your GED while looking for a job. Start moving in the right direction. Both you and your child deserve it. I am distressed because I know you are a smart young woman. In life, what separates the successes and the failures is the ability of the former to hone the skills and talents with which they have been blessed. I am here to help you, if you decide I could assist in any of your positive endeavors.

I look forward to hearing from you soon. Bye for now and God bless you and your child.

Sincerely,

Ngozi Osuagwu, MD, FACOG

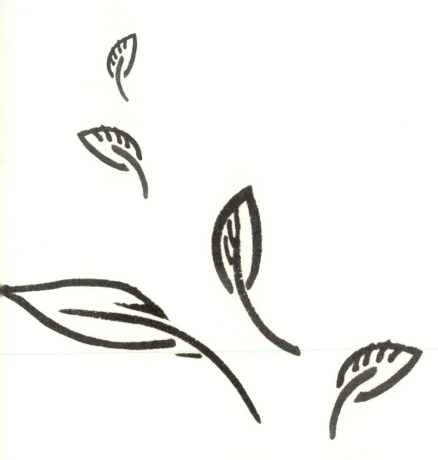

It is easier to rule a kingdom
than to regulate a family.

 JAPANESE PROVERB

Dear Carmen,

Thank you for sharing your story last night during the meeting of the Women's Network. I know that you are going through a lot, but I am very concerned. I have known you for six years and during that time, you have gained seventy-five pounds. You have now been diagnosed with hypertension and your primary care physician (PCP) is monitoring you for diabetes. I am especially concerned because I know that your children are your number one priority. But if you don't take care of yourself, you won't be around for your children.

You have to find time to take care of yourself. You must come first in your life. When you told me about the stresses in your life, the first thing that came to my mind was this has to change. Make positive changes in your life and count your blessings. The solution is not eating fast food, remaining sedentary, or moping about your rotten luck.

The fact is that you have a wonderful family. I see many patients who are struggling to have children and are willing to do almost anything to have a child, yet you have three children. You have a husband, so you don't have the struggles and travails of most single moms. You have a job and live in a decent neighborhood with an excellent school system.

I know you would love to stay at home and raise your children; unfortunately you cannot afford it. You would love to have your children in every after school activity, but you don't have the time. You want your husband to help you more around the house, but he is working three jobs just to afford to live in the neighborhood with the good school systems.

We all want things that we may not be able to get, but you are putting too much stress on yourself about it. For you to come up with some solutions, you need quiet time for yourself. Find ten minutes either in the morning or the evening just to be alone. Take time to breathe deeply and appreciate life. I have found that starting out this way, you begin to find more time to do other things.

I am not sure if you know that I have been practicing yoga for some years and it has really helped me take care of me. By taking care of me, I have been able to take care of my loved ones better. My husband is always quick to remind me that the flight attendants always ask that you get your own oxygen mask on before turning to help anyone else. While it may sound selfish, you are much more valuable to everyone else when you have taken care of yourself.

Sincerely,

Ngozi Osuagwu, MD, FACOG

Somehow we must get across to our
daughters, sisters and best friends that
while being in a relationship can be
wonderful and healthy, depending solely
on others to define ourselves is limiting
and unfulfilling.

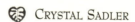 CRYSTAL SADLER

Dear Christine,

I don't understand why you don't get it. You have been with your boyfriend for the past four years and you inform me in that time you have never been unfaithful. Yet, I have diagnosed you with chlamydia twice and gonorrhea once in this same period. Yesterday, I told you that your cultures came back positive for herpes. Before you start those funny questions, these sexually transmitted infections do not come from public toilet seats or sharing towels. Unfortunately, while the chlamydia and gonorrhea are completely treatable because they are bacterial infections, it is not the case with herpes. In the case of herpes, only the symptoms can be managed.

What is the problem? How can I help you? How about some love with your eyes open? Yes, I know a "good man" is hard to find, but is the man infecting you with sexually transmitted infections really a good man? My husband will sometimes tell me that one story is true until you hear the other side. I hope I am not making an ass of myself by believing you that he is the straying partner. Yeah, it may be easier for me to be self-righteous because I have a mate. Yeah, I can't hold my toy and tell it I love it like I can with a man. But, I tell you I will use one of the many toys readily available to get my pleasure, if it is what is absolutely necessary, rather than staying with a man who infects me with all kinds of diseases. I have patients who swear the pleasure even surpasses what men can do. Have I had a first-hand experience? The answer is simply no.

I know you "love" your boyfriend, but it is time that both of you have an open discussion about your relationship. It is time that you ask the hard questions—of him and of yourself. If you want and it makes it easier for you, you can bring him to the next office visit so that we can go over the results together and I can help both of you start a frank discussion about your relationship. I hasten to add that I am not a psychologist and further exploration of your relationship will have to be handled by those who are trained to handle such matters. As I tell my husband all the time, my specialty is restricted to the area between the belly button and the knee in women. Please call the office and schedule the appointment.

Sincerely,

Ngozi Osuagwu, MD, FACOG

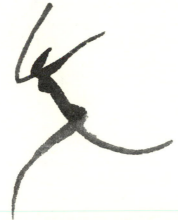

I can't remember what I was doing before running. I guess shopping, sewing, watching TV—gaining nothing.

MIKI GORMAN, MARATHON RUNNER

Dear Lauren,

You are twenty one years old and weigh three hundred and sixty-five pounds. I don't know what has happened. In a single year, you gained forty-five pounds. Don't you listen to all the news on obesity? How do I tell you that what you are doing is wrong? Stop making excuses and take charge of the situation. You say you are old enough to date. Yet when I asked you what you plan to do about your weight, you told me you are waiting for your mother. I was unclear and remain so about what you meant by replying that you are waiting for your mother.

I couldn't help but also notice that you weren't in the mood to listen to what I had to say. You were in a hurry and simply wanted me to give you a prescription. It seems that, like many people, you want a magic bullet. They want me to give them a pill or tell them something profound. The fact is you need to believe there is something wrong and that you have a problem with food. The basic way to lose weight is to take in less and get out more. If you are really serious about losing weight, you need to think about what you eat, when you eat, and why you eat. The road does not stop there; this goes beyond diet. You also need to believe that you can do something to help yourself. You can buy all the diet books in the world, but nothing is going to help if you don't start moving. Exercise! Exercise! Exercise! Do anything but not nothing; it can be walking, running, yoga, Pilates®. It can be Tae Bo®, swimming, or dancing. The possibilities are endless.

Do you know that if the American people ate their five servings of fruits and vegetables a day, the cancer rate would decrease by forty percent? I am not saying that you should stop eating sweets and those things that make life so pleasurable; rather, you should limit them. Think about all those late night snacks. Are they necessary? Should you eat when you are angry or experiencing any other strong emotion? It is all about choices.

I hope you take what I say to heart. Yes, you might get upset, but I am your physician, and remember, the hallmark of my practice is open and honest communication. I would be failing in my responsibilities to you as a physician if I did not inform you that you are obese and on a dangerous path to ill health. I don't want to see you forty-five pounds heavier the next time you come in to the office, and I certainly do not want you saying I failed to inform you of the dangers of obesity if you find yourself in a dialysis center in the future. I can always pull out and re-read this letter and satisfy my conscience that I warned you even though privacy laws prevent me from sharing it with the world.

Sincerely,

Ngozi Osuagwu, MD, FACOG

It's not the men in my life that
counts—it's the life in my men.

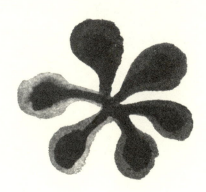 MAE WEST

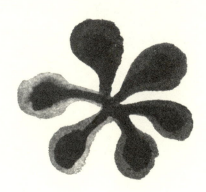

Dear Ms. Riddle,

It was quite refreshing to hear you reply, "I'm not dead yet," in response to my inquiry regarding your sex life. At seventy-four, it is a good thing that you still have a healthy sexual appetite. I am writing to you about my observation that you were very uncomfortable discussing your husband's current condition with him. If he is having problems sustaining an erection and pleasing you sexually, he needs to seek help. In most cases, there are options available to him to be able to perform this very important husbandly duty.

I also don't want you to feel embarrassed in any of our discussions. I would like you to be comfortable and forthright. Rarely have I come across an issue or problem that I have not encountered before, and believe me, your problem is not isolated. While I am not a sexologist, I can make some suggestions and/or refer you to a specialist.

Try to initiate a conversation with your husband; in your conversation, suggest that he see a physician. There are many drugs available to help men sustain an erection. His problems may be related to some of his prescription medications. He needs to be honest with his physician about his symptoms and about any medications he is taking.

It is not abnormal to seek sexual gratification with your hands or devices. You should, however, talk to your husband, because this is an issue that affects both of you. Why should women suffer in silence? Often, when women have sexual problems, men seek gratification outside the relationship. Women need to be vocal and tell their partners about what they like and do not like. If we are not being pleased by them sexually, we need to communicate it clearly, and not be demure and suffer in silence. Men cannot read our minds. They need to understand that our bodies are dynamic entities with changing requirements and responses.

Your husband's condition is not uncommon and routinely affects men with diabetes or prostrate problems. It may also be because of other problems. Sometimes it is the difficulty with erections that alert physicians to other medical problems. Suggest and implore him to see a doctor. Accompany him to his doctor's office and help with questions that he is uncomfortable asking.

I also have books that I can lend you. Please do stop by the office and borrow one of my books on tips to start the conversation with your husband. If it helps, have him accompany you to my office, and we can initiate a conversation here that hopefully will produce some answers that guide us on what steps to take in resolving the issues that concern you.

Sincerely,

Ngozi Osuagwu, MD, FACOG

What we have to do is to find
a way to celebrate our
diversity and debate our
differences without
fracturing our communities.

HILLARY RODHAM CLINTON

Make peace with the fact that
you are not always going to be
able to do everything people
will ask of you.

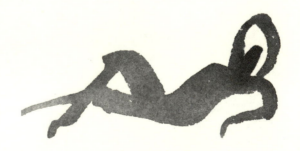 VALERIE FERGUSON

Dear Ria,

What kind of physician will I be if I let this situation continue to fester? How can a friend be a victim of domestic violence and I am oblivious to it? Can I ever sleep again if anything happens to you, and I was privy to this secret and did nothing about it? I cannot continue to fool myself. I am going to report my suspicion that you are being physically abused to the authorities for investigation. I wanted to let you know in advance so that we could talk.

I have known you and your husband for the past 4 years. I never suspected what was happening since your marriage seemed so perfect. I even teased my husband and told him that he should be more like Peter. I was so happy when I found out you were pregnant and honored when you chose to see me for your prenatal care. The first day you came to my office for care, I noted the bruise on your abdomen. You told me you fell down and I had no reason to doubt you. You were about 12 weeks pregnant at that time. I had no reason to check you again until you complained of vaginal itching at 24 weeks. Your left thigh was scalded. It was one of the worse burns I have seen. You told me it was the result of a cooking accident, although the presentation of the burn was not consistent with how you described the accident.

You are now 32 weeks. When you complained of vaginal bleeding, I became very concerned. The ER physician called me knowing that you were a friend of mine. She informed me of the bruises she noticed on your back. She told me that you told her that you fell and that I was aware of the situation. You told her that you were with me when you fell. Your lie to the ER doctor made it all come together for me. Wow! You are the victim of spousal physical abuse. Since all your visits to the hospital were documented in the hospital's computer systems, I went over the records of your ER visits and was shocked. The dates of your ER visits coincided to the dates your husband had told me that you were visiting your relatives. I will be failing in my responsibilities to you and the unborn child if I do not report it immediately.

This decision did not come easy. I know that you might not want to talk to me again, but I can't take the chance of something happening to you or worse yet, something happening to your unborn child. I went online and conducted a search for Hedda Nussbaum and asked you to read about her. I did it with the hope you can begin to understand why I have decided to alerts the agencies better equipped and trained than me to deal with the problem of domestic violence. Why did I fool myself believing that domestic violence is restricted to people in the lower socio-economic classes? How could I stay oblivious to your private mayhem and public mirth for a long time?

I decided to give you this letter in my office, and fortunately, during this appointment, work issues prevented him from coming along. Please read this letter and have it shredded before leaving my office. I am sure you know my reasons. We can talk some more if you wish, but I have already informed the professionals at Columbus Coalition against Family Violence and they have a counselor who will talk with you as soon as your prenatal visit is over, unless you choose not to, against my medical advice.

Sincerely,

Ngozi Osuagwu, MD, FACOG

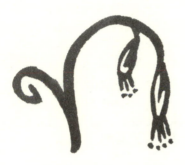

For happiness one needs security, but joy can spring like a flower even from the cliffs of despair.

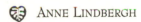 ANNE LINDBERGH

Dear Miki,

I can't begin to know how you feel, but I know it must be hard. When you found out early in your pregnancy that you were going to have a baby with severe cardiac defects, I wondered what you would do. Most importantly, I did not want to bring in any of my biases. I knew you had one healthy child at home, and I wanted to make sure that you understood the full ramifications of continuing the pregnancy. The baby would need surgery at birth, and there was no guarantee that the baby would survive the procedure. You would probably be in and out of the hospital for the rest of the child's life. I wondered how that would affect your family life: would you have time for the child at home?

I knew that as your physician I would have to discuss all of the options with you. One would be to keep the child, and the other would be to abort. I had a good idea of what my decision would be if I were in the same situation. Then I remembered that I am just your physician; I am not God. Yes, God gave me a wonderful gift, but I was not God. I decided to pray for you. I prayed to God to help you make a good decision.

Once you decided to go through with the pregnancy, I decided mentally that I would stand behind you. I saw what the future could be, and I continued to pray. I prayed for you and your husband and I prayed for the little one at home. I watched your abdomen grow and I continued to pray that God would continue to guide you. All the specialists said everything was okay, and I continued to pray.

Then you made that phone call. You had not felt the baby move for a whole day. I knew then that things were not good. I sent you to the hospital, but I think we both knew what they would find. The ultrasound showed no fetal movement and showed no heart beat. I gave you your options; either we could let things happen on their own or I could induce labor. You decided to stay to have labor induced and get delivered.

What I could not tell you was that it was all very hard for me. I don't do well delivering babies that are stillborn. I prayed that the baby would look normal. I prayed that I would not faint. I was scared, but I knew I had to be strong. After all, you had made a strong decision to proceed with the pregnancy. The next morning you delivered and I was there. I watched you and your husband cry. Somehow, I knew this was best. The next day you went home. The next time I heard from you was when you requested the autopsy report and a copy of your chart.

I still pray for you. I hope that you find the strength to move on. I wish I could have been there for a live birth, but such was not the case. I just wanted to write to tell you that I care. Best wishes with the next doctor and the next pregnancy. Please continue to pray.

Sincerely

Ngozi Osuagwu, MD, FACOG

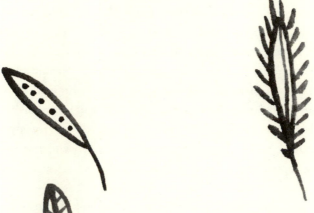

One of the best lessons children learn through video games is standing still will get them killed quicker than anything else.

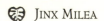 JINX MILEA

Dear Patricia,

I am sorry I have not gotten back to you. I don't understand why you continue to stay with a physician with whom you have difficulty talking. Am I missing something? Your physicians cannot help you if you do not talk to them. As I have always told my patients, "medical school taught me many things, but it did not teach me how to read minds."

Yes, you were sent in to see me for evaluation of an abnormal pap smear, but I cannot in good conscience ignore your other problems. You have hypertension and it is not being controlled at this time. You told me that you saw your physician last month and your blood pressure was 160/100. Today your blood pressure is 180/100. In healthy people, normal blood pressure is 120/80. The higher number is the systolic pressure, which represents the maximum pressure in your arteries when you exert energy. The lower number is the diastolic pressure; it represents the pressure when your heart is at rest. Both of your readings are well above the normal level and present a serious risk to your health. You cannot ignore this problem anymore. You need medication to get your blood pressure under control. Hypertension has been dubbed the silent killer because it can lead to other fatal conditions including stroke, heart failure, heart attack, kidney failure, and vision problems without the individual knowing they are sick.

You can diet, cut down on your salt intake, and increase exercise, but above all, you need medication to get your blood pressure under control immediately. I can't understand the problem. You must take control of your health. You need to learn more about your condition and discuss the issue with your primary care physician. It is your health and life. You can't be bashful or afraid of talking to your internist about the problems that I have definitely diagnosed. Cardiovascular disease kills more women each year than all forms of cancer.

Since you came to me for follow-up on an abnormal Pap smear, let us discuss that problem. As I informed you during your last visit, we performed a colposcopy, a procedure where I used an instrument called the colposcope to better visualize your cervix. During the colposcopy, I took some samples of the cervix from the area where I felt was the cause of the abnormality of the Pap smear. These samples were sent to the lab for testing that will tell us what is causing the abnormality.

I am still waiting for the test results on the samples I obtained during the colposcopy, and my office will call you as soon as we have it. I chose to send this letter because I feel that your blood pressure represents a greater concern that needs immediate attention. Please follow up quickly with your primary care doctor. If your doctor does not have time for you, then it is time for you to consider finding another one.

Sincerely,

Ngozi Osuagwu, MD, FACOG

Healthy families have a rule that
each family member can honestly
say what they experience and ask
for what they want.

VIRGINIA SATIR

Dear Lila,

When I saw that you scheduled an appointment for a pregnancy test, I was surprised. I have known you for seven years and you have never mentioned any thing about a man in your life. In the medical history you provided to my nurse, and during our discussions, you always stated that you were not sexually active, only for us to find out you are now pregnant. Is this man a new one, or has he been lurking in the shadows because you did not want to tell me you were with a married man?

Well, I can see why you did not want to talk about him; the circumstances are interesting, but not unique. The man is married and has three children. He wants you to have an abortion. I can see that you were not thrilled with that option. I discussed adoption, but you did not appear to like that idea either. In that case, we are really left with only one option. You keep the baby and raise him or her the best way you can. It won't be easy, but I think you will feel better going that route.

You did not come to my office to be judged, and I want it to be clear that I am not making any judgment on your choices. My primary responsibility is to take care of your healthcare needs. However, if we are going to continue our patient-doctor relationship, it has to be one based on open and frank communication. Being selective in providing information about your medical history cannot allow me to have the complete picture of your medical conditions that is necessary to make the best medical calls to take care of you. And I have to suggest we begin a new relationship, one based on complete trust and honesty. If we cannot have a relationship where I can get your complete history, I may miss a diagnosis and get into trouble.

Unless you assure me that you are being forthright, you may have to look for a new physician. I am enclosing another copy of the patient history form for you to complete for your files in my office. Completing it over the course of some time will enable you to remember most of the information being requested in the form.

I hope to see you regardless of your decision about your pregnancy. If you are uncertain about which direction to go with respect to the pregnancy, I do suggest that you start taking multivitamins. These will benefit both you and the baby if you decide to go forward with your pregnancy. If you choose to keep the baby, or have it and put the child for adoption, please contact my office to schedule an initial prenatal visit. If abortion is the path you choose, you already have a list of doctors who can perform the procedure. Let me know how you choose to proceed.

Sincerely,

Ngozi Osuagwu, MD, FACOG

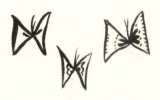

Treatment is truly a cooperative
effort of a trinity——the patient,
the doctor, and the inner doctor.

RALPH BIRCHER

Dear Katie,

I am so sorry that I did not take you more seriously. Physicians often call people like you "frequent flyers." You were always in my office, but because you refused my suggestions that we do an exploratory surgery to find out the cause of the pain, I was beginning to doubt you and was wondering whether you were only coming to the office because you wanted pain medication. I was actually beginning to feel that I had a problem with someone addicted to pain medications. After two years, I am glad you finally decided to have the diagnostic laparoscopy, a procedure where I insert a telescope-like instrument through a small incision to take a look inside your abdomen and try to determine what may be causing your pain.

The good news is that I have found the cause of your pain. You have severe endometriosis. Endometriosis occurs when cells that usually line your uterus are found outside the uterus. These cells can be found on your ovaries, the fallopian tubes, and the bowels, as well as other tissues. Endometriosis can cause chronic pain. Your pain has been unbearable because these cells were also growing inside your ovaries and fallopian tubes. During the diagnostic laparoscopy I noted that you had scar tissue everywhere in your reproductive system. I could not even move your ovaries.

The bad news is that the endometriosis was so severe that it may affect your fertility in the future. I removed as much as I could during the surgery. I would like to see you soon to discuss the options for managing your endometriosis and stopping further progression of the disease. Please schedule an appointment soon.

Sincerely,

Ngozi Osuagwu, MD FACOG

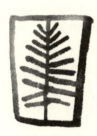

A woman is like a teabag; you never know how strong she is until she gets in hot water.

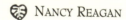 NANCY REAGAN

Dear Chelsea,

How many times must I tell you that you do not have to douche? Douching removes the vaginal flora and alters the balance of microorganisms in your vagina. By douching and washing away most of the good bacteria, you increase the dominance of the bad bacteria, which creates the vaginitis that brings you to my office. Douching is not good for you, unless it is your way of supporting my practice. My preference would be for you to support my practice by refering your friends.

It is not unusual for women to have a mild discharge. In fact, the discharge is a result of the vagina cleaning itself. Let me put it this way; just as the saliva that forms in our mouth during the day keeps the mouth relatively clean, the discharge from the vagina keeps the vagina clean. The only difference between the vagina and the mouth is that we swallow the saliva, but the discharge drains out.

Normally most women have vaginal discharge, which keeps the vagina moist and clean. This discharge should be clear or white. When it dries, it may leave a yellowish color on your underpants. Some women halfway between periods may have a few days of clear, heavy, and slippery vaginal discharge, which occurs when the one of the ovaries releases a ripe egg.

If you notice a vaginal discharge that is unusual from your normal discharge, it is important to schedule an appointment. This is to make a definitive diagnosis of your condition. The doctor may need to obtain a sample and examine it under a microscope to determine the cause of the discharge and the best treatment for you. Common vaginal infections are trichomoniasis, candidiasis, bacterial vaginosis, and atrophic vaginitis.

If you have any of the following symptoms, it is an indication you have a vaginal infection and should see me or another doctor if you are not in Columbus.

- Change in vaginal discharge
- Itching or burning around the vagina
- Painful Intercourse
- Chills or Fevers
- Abdominal Pain or Cramping
- Burning when you urinate
- Sores or warts near the vaginal opening.

Of course, it is always wise to take care of yourself and follow practices that help prevent infections. There are ways to prevent vaginal infections:

- Stay healthy, exercise regularly, eat balanced meals, and get some rest.
- Keep yourself clean and wipe from front to back.
- Do not wear tight-fitting undergarments and clothing.
- Stay away from irritating chemicals like bubble baths and douching products.
- Use condoms during sexual intercourse to protect yourself from sexually transmitted diseases.

I hope I have given you a good discourse of vaginal discharge. If you believe you have an infection and/or have additional questions, please call the office and schedule an appointment to see me. Thank you.

Sincerely,

Ngozi Osuagwu, MD, FACOG

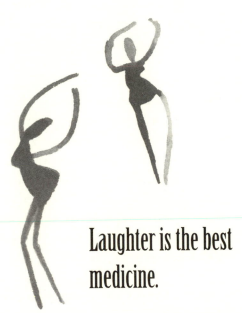

Laughter is the best medicine.

🌿 PROVERB

Dear Hawa,

This letter is being written to explain again why I switched your medicines. Although we discussed the reasons for the change during your visit to the office, I noticed a puzzled expression on your face as I left the examination room. While it was not immediately apparent to me, on my reflection at the end of the day, I felt that it may be necessary to further explain the reasons, hence this letter.

Medicines work differently in men and women. Hormones can influence the way medicines work in our bodies and because the levels of hormones in a woman's body varies, medication level can also vary. There are medicines, which we can normally prescribe for you, but will not do so if you are pregnant because it can cause problems for the unborn child. We can also change medications or the dosages we prescribe, as you age, because older women process medicines differently from younger women, in part due to the changes in hormone levels.

If you have completed the patient history form, you will notice in bold letters the section that asks whether you are allergic to any medicine. The question is in bold letters because it is important for your doctor to know which medicines could cause a potentially serious reaction. Since I am obstetrician/gynecologist, if you plan to get pregnant, or are already pregnant, I need to know. It is also important to ask any other doctor or me certain questions about any medication that is prescribed for you: what symptoms or condition is it meant to treat; are there side effects of which you should be aware and about the safety of taking the prescribed medicine with other medicines and supplements. You should also find out the right way to take the medicine, whether it is a good idea to drive after taking this medicine, and whether you should avoid certain drinks like alcohol and caffeinated drinks when taking the medicine.

Keep a list of prescriptions you receive and the time you started taking each one. Always review the list with your doctor and pharmacist during every visit. You also need to let the doctor know immediately if you start having symptoms that you did not have prior to taking the new medicine. Finally, it is important to know that no question is a dumb question as far as medicine, or for that matter, food that you ingest.

I changed your medicine because you informed me that you and your husband were trying to have a baby. There are different classes of medicines for the management of your condition and I decided to change your prescription and give you medicine that is not likely to impact the development of your child when you conceive. The new medicine may not work as well as the old one; however, it is safer for your unborn child should you become pregnant. I hope I have explained my reasons for changing your medicine fairly clearly.

Sincerely,

Ngozi Osuagwu, MD, FACOG

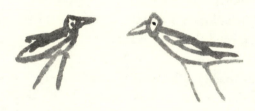

Don't compromise yourself.
You are all you've got.

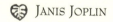 JANIS JOPLIN

Dear Yvonne,

I am so glad that you decided to come home to practice Law. It
has been delightful watching you grow from a precocious teenager
to the Editor of your law school journal, and now the highly
touted and most sought lawyer of your law school class. I am
impressed and very happy for you and your parents. The last time
I saw you was just before you went off to Law School. You are so
grown up now. Soon I will be holding you to your promise to give
me free legal advice.

I am equally excited about this new person you met. Based on
how you describe him, he is definitely better than your boyfriend
from college. "A woman has got to love a bad man once or twice
in her life to be thankful for a good one"—Marjorie Kinnan
Rawlings. As you told me during your visit, you haven't been in
an intimate relationship since you broke up with the guy from
your college days. You did the right thing to come in for your
annual. I went ahead and performed a pap smear and obtained
cultures for gonorrhea and chlamydia. I should have your results
back in a few weeks. You mentioned that he is seeing his doctor
as well. Is it just for a routine physical?

You declined to get tested for human immunodeficiency virus
(HIV). I hope that you are not offended by the fact I brought it
up. The disease is real. Real people have the disease. You cannot
look at a person and tell that they have the virus. My making the
suggestion to get tested does not in any way imply that you
engaged in any high-risk behavior likely to have exposed you to
the virus. I was not implying any such thing of your new
boyfriend either. All I am saying is that in this day and age, it is
not unreasonable to suggest that both of you should get tested

and know your status. The results need not change anything about your relationship, but at least you go into it after full disclosure by both people involved.

You are forcing me to share my own history, and I do so only because I hope it helps make me more credible and elucidate my reason for making my suggestion. When I started dating my husband, then my boyfriend, he was concerned. Although, I didn't have the obvious risk factors for HIV, he was concerned because as an ob-gyn doctor I deal with bodily fluids all the time. I still remind him of the retort from his cousin, a nephrologist, when he brought up the issue of possible exposure to the disease. His cousin told him to leave the kitchen if he could not deal with the heat. Doctors will always support their colleagues, even against their cousins. I was not opposed to testing, especially after he made it clear that for him it was necessary to get the test to take our relationship to the next level, which was marriage. I also wanted to know, so we made our appointment and went together to the health department. Waiting for the results was probably one of the stressful times of my life, but the happiness of getting the negative result made it all worthwhile. 15 years later, I am very careful, while working in the hospital setting.

You and your boyfriend need to make your next date at the Health Department. Get a blood test for HIV. While you are there, also get a blood test for herpes. Both of you should know your status. I am not saying it should prevent you from seeing each other, but at least you would know the necessary precautions to take in case one of you tests positive. If you stayed celibate for three years in Law School, avoiding intercourse for a couple of weeks ought not make any difference in your relationship with this new beau.

Yvonne, I am so proud of all your accomplishments. Watching your transformation has given me a sense of what I hope to see as my daughters grow up. I have been you doctor since you came to me for your first gynecologic exam immediately after your first period, and I have watched you grow to an extraordinary woman. I am sure that you know I am not a cynic, although there's no escaping the label of being a realist. I am sure you know I would never give you any advice I would not give my own daughters. Be good. If you need to talk some more, do give me a call.

Sincerely,

Ngozi Osuagwu, MD, FACOG

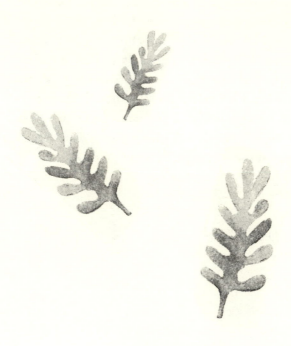

Without faith, nothing is possible.
With it, nothing is impossible.

 Mary McLeod Bethune

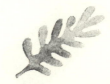

Dear Zoe,

I apologize if you found the tone of my letter offensive. It was not my intention to offend you, however I do not believe in sugar coating matters. You are my sister, since you have entrusted me with caring for your health. I would be doing you a disservice, if I did not speak with you truthfully, even if I was a little blunt. If you felt I criticized you, it was only supposed to be of a constructive variety. However, I do appreciate your honesty for bringing up your feelings, and I am glad you did not go looking for another doctor because of the tone of my letter.

I am flattered you asked me to tell you how I take care of myself. It is pertinent to mention that you have to find your own way and what works for you. I start my morning with a contemplative prayer while lying on my bed. After brushing my teeth, it is either a session of Yoga or Pilates. If it is a short session, I incorporate some cardiovascular exercise by riding my stationary bike. A shower and mandatory breakfast, even if it is on the go, are essential for me to have a productive day at work. During the warm months, I'll walk three miles two or three days of the week. In exercise, I have found consistency to be very helpful.

Since I truly enjoy food and have a knee-buckling weakness for some richer ones, when I indulge, I compensate by spending more time on my exercises. I eat a lot of vegetables and supplement with vitamins. For more reasons than one, I read the labels of food items I buy and I am very selective about the choices I make. Occasionally, I will drink some wine and cocktails on social occasions. I do not smoke or indulge in street or psychedelic drugs. I also try to avoid anyone who smokes or uses drugs.

I always get my routine physicals—Pap smear, mammogram, colorectal screening, dental checks, and vision checks. I will soon incorporate dermatologic visits. It is a good idea to do your monthly breast examinations, although this is an area where I have truly not been as diligent as I should. Even though I am doctor, I also have to learn about health issues that affect me, which means I am a voracious reader of materials in integrative medicine. I am vigilant about the changes in my body, but not overly obsessive about it.

I find reading, learning about new things, and keeping a journal very rewarding. It is very interesting to pick up my journal and read about things I wrote years ago. I am not very good at making new friends, but I keep trying. Having said that, I do have many good friends that have transcended into sisters. I find that I like speaking about health and healthcare, and when opportunities to do so are present, I will often volunteer. I find fulfillment in sharing my experiences and interacting with my audience and gaining new insights very rewarding.

Central to my being is my relationship with the Almighty, for whom I am only an instrument. My life and my relationships are guided by my faith and in my every action, I try to express love, sometimes in tough doses, but always guided by the desire to do good. Am I fallible? Yes, you bet. Do I keep trying to be a better person? Sure, I do. Am I above being reproached? No.

My life is in perfect harmony when I am able to keep these dimensions balanced – physical, mental, spiritual, social, domestic and financial. I sincerely believe that if you are able to balance these aspects of life, you will always be happy. I hope I have answered your question. The path I outlined in this letter is mine. You have to choose yours. In doing so, you may choose to use aspects of what I do. Once again, thank you for being honest and telling me how you feel. I hope your annoyance is tempered by the fact that any comments I made were for your benefit. If you have any more comments and/or questions, please do not hesitate to contact me.

Sincerely,

Ngozi Osuagwu, MD, FACOG

PS: My patients over forty always told me it is very difficult to stay trim. Don't I know it now? My ability to fight back is helped now only because I developed the habit of exercising when I was younger. Does that mean you cannot start an exercise program now? No.

Character contributes to beauty. It
fortifies a woman as her youth fades.
A mode of conduct, a standard of
courage, discipline, fortitude, and
integrity can do a great deal to make
a woman beautiful.

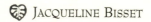 JACQUELINE BISSET

Common Gynecologic Conditions

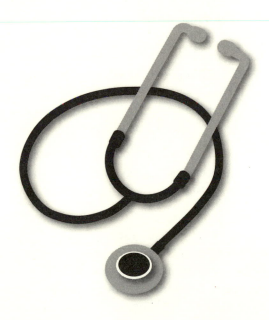

A number of gynecologic conditions send women to their obste-
trician/gynecologist. In this section, we discuss some of the
conditions and the parts of the female anatomy affected by each.
The list is not exhaustive but includes the majority of common
conditions, as identified by the American College of Obstetricians
and Gynecologists in its Fact Book for 2004. Following the
description of each condition is a list of websites where you can
find more information.

Dysmenorrhea

Primary dysmenorrhea, also known as menstrual pain, affects a
significant percentage of young women in their teens and early
twenties. The pain usually starts a day or two before menstrual
flow and may continue through the first two days of menstruation.
It is believed that this pain is the leading cause of recurrent short-
term school absence in adolescent girls. The discomfort experi-
enced by women tends to decrease over time and after pregnancy.
Underlying physical problems cause secondary dysmenorrhea.

The American College of Obstetricians and Gynecologists states
that about three quarters of women experience primary dysmenorrhea, and fifteen percent have reported having severe menstrual
cramps.

http://www.umm.edu/altmed/ConsConditions/Dysmenorrheacc.html
http://www.health.umd.edu/Library/Handouts/dysmen.pdf
http://www.aafp.org/afp/20050115/285.html

Ectopic Pregnancy

An ectopic pregnancy occurs when the fertilized egg attaches itself in
a place other than inside the uterus; most commonly, an egg will

attach in the fallopian tubes. Since only the uterus is designed to properly accommodate a growing embryo, and the potential for rupture and hemorrhage always exists in an ectopic pregnancy. Early prenatal care and ultrasonography can identify this type of pregnancy before it becomes life threatening. Ruptured ectopic pregnancies are the leading cause for maternal mortality in the first trimester and account for about 10 percent of all pregnancy-related deaths.

Some women will still have menstrual like bleeding during pregnancy. It is important to pay attention to the flow, because decreased flow along with some pain may be indicative of an ectopic pregnancy, if you are sexually active. A physician should be contacted immediately to evaluate the symptoms to rule out ectopic pregnancy.

http://www.americanpregnancy.org/pregnancycomplications/ectopicpregnancy.html
http://kidshealth.org/parent/pregnancy_newborn/pregnancy/ectopic.html
http://www.nlm.nih.gov/medlineplus/ency/article/000895.htm

Endometriosis

Endometriosis occurs when the tissue that lines the uterus, called endometrium, grows outside of the uterus. This tissue as it grows can develop into tumors that cause pain, irregular periods, heavy bleeding, and often lead to infertility. Most times, severe pelvic pain affects women with endometriosis during their monthly menstrual cycle. Besides the uterus, endometriosis may also occur in other places in the female organs. Endometriosis can occur in the ovaries and the fallopian tubes. Endometriosis to a lesser extent has also been found in the vagina, inside the bladder, bowels, intestines, and on scars from previous surgeries

http://www.4woman.gov/faq/endomet.pdf
http://www.americanpregnancy.org/womenshealth/endometriosis.html
http://www.endometriosis.org/endometriosis.html

Osteoporosis

Osteoporosis, which literally means "porous bones," is a disease in which bones become progressively weak, brittle, and more likely to break. It is characterized by a progressive loss of bone density, thinning bone tissue, and increased likelihood of fracture. Left untreated, osteoporosis can progress silently and painlessly until the breakage of a bone. A seemingly symptom-less disease, it is often undetected until a bump or fall causes fractures or a vertebra collapses resulting in back pain. Osteoporosis overwhelmingly affects women—especially Caucasian women—over the age of fifty-five, but it also occurs in men and can occur at any age.

http://www.osteoporosisinfo.org
http://www.nlm.nih.gov/medlineplus/osteoporosis.html
http://www.nof.org

Pelvic Inflammatory Disease (PID)

Pelvic inflammatory disease (PID) is a general term that refers to infection of upper genital tract—the uterus, fallopian tubes, and other parts of the reproductive organ. It is one of the most common and serious complications of sexually transmitted diseases (STDs) like chlamydia and gonorrhea. PID can cause scarring and lead to infertility, ectopic pregnancy, and chronic pelvic discomfort.

http://www.medinfo.co.uk/conditions/pid.html
http://www.cdc.gov/std/PID/STDFact-PID.htm
http://www.nlm.nih.gov/medlineplus/pelvicinflammatorydisease.html

Polycystic ovary syndrome (PCOS)

Polycystic ovary syndrome (PCOS) is a disorder in which normal hormone cycles are disrupted causing irregular reproductive function in women of childbearing age. Enlarged ovaries with small cysts and a high number of follicles characterize polycystic ovary syndrome at various stages of maturation. Women with PCOS are likely to have high levels of male hormones (androgens), resulting in increased hair on the face, back, and chest. PCOS can also cause irregular or no menstrual cycle and affect fertility, hormones, insulin production, heart, blood vessels, and appearance.

http://www.4woman.gov/faq/pcos.htm
http://www.pcosupport.org

Urinary tract infection (UTI)

Urinary tract infections (often referred to by its acronym UTI) occur when microorganisms, usually bacteria from the digestive tract, cling to the opening of the urethra and begin to multiply. Most infections can be attributed to the *E. coli* bacteria that normally live in the colon. There are three main types of UTI: urethritis (urethra), cystitis (bladder), and pyelonephritis (kidney). A bacterial urinary tract infection is the most common kind of infection affecting the urinary tract. UTIs cause discomfort and the frequent urge to urinate accompanied by a burning sensation.

http://kidshealth.org/teen/sexual_health/stds/uti.html
www.pueblo.gsa.gov/cic_text/health/urinarytract/utiadult.htm
http://kidney.niddk.nih.gov/kudiseases/pubs/utiadult/

Uterine Fibroids

Uterine fibroids are tumors made up of muscle cells and other tissues that grow within the wall of the uterus (or womb). The growths are almost always benign (not cancerous). Fibroids can grow as a single growth or in clusters. Their size can vary from that of a coin to even larger than a grapefruit. An estimated 20-50 percent of women of childbearing age have uterine fibroids.

Fibroids are known in some cases to affect childbearing ability of some women.

www.4woman.gov/faq/fibroids.pdf
http://www.uterine-fibroids.org/about-uterine-fibroids.html
http://www.mayoclinic.com/health/uterine-fibroids/DS00078
http://www.nichd.nih.gov/publications/pubs/fibroids/index.htm

Yeast Infection

An organism known as *Candida albicans* causes vaginal yeast infections. Normally, small numbers of these tiny organisms inhabit the skin and live inside the vagina. The normal acidic environment of the vagina helps keep yeast from multiplying. When the fungus overgrows in the vagina, a yeast infection develops, causing uncomfortable symptoms such as vaginal itching, burning, and discharge. In the course of their lifetime, at least seventy-five percent of women will have at least one vaginal yeast infection. The pH balance of the vagina can change because of your period (menstruation), pregnancy, diabetes, some antibiotics, birth control pills, and steroids. Moisture and irritation of the vagina also seem to encourage yeast to grow.

http://familydoctor.org/206.xml
http://www.healthywomen.org/content.cfm?L1=3&L2=93
http://www.nlm.nih.gov/medlineplus/ency/article/001511.htm

Sexually Transmitted Diseases

If you have sex, you may be at risk for a sexually transmitted disease. Your chances of becoming infected increases if:

- You or your partner has or had other sexual partners;
- You do not always use condoms consistently and correctly;
- Your partner has a sexually transmitted disease;
- You use injection drugs; or
- You exchange sex for money or drugs.

The most common sexually transmitted diseases or STDs in the United States are:

Chlamydia

Chlamydia is a common sexually transmitted disease caused by the bacterium *chlamydia trachomatis*, which can damage a woman's reproductive organs. Chlamydia infection can occur during oral, vaginal, or anal sexual contact with an infected partner. Even though symptoms of chlamydia are usually mild or absent, serious complications that cause irreversible damage, including infertility, can occur "silently" before a woman ever recognizes a problem. It is also associated with pelvic inflammatory disease (PID). Chlamydia also can cause discharge from the penis of an infected man. It is estimated by The Centers for Disease Control and Prevention (CDC) that more than three million people are infected each year.

http://www.niaid.nih.gov/factsheets/stdclam.htm
http://www.cdc.gov/std/chlamydia/STDFact-chlamydia.htm
http://www.4woman.gov/faq/stdchlam.htm

Gonorrhea

Gonorrhea is a sexually transmitted disease (STD). Gonorrhea is caused by *Neisseria gonorrhoeae*, a bacterium that can grow and multiply easily in the warm, moist areas of the reproductive tract, including the cervix (opening to the womb), uterus (womb), and fallopian tubes (egg canals) in women, and in the urethra (urine canal) in women and men. In women, this disease can spread into the uterus and fallopian tubes, resulting in pelvic inflammatory disease (PID).

According to CDC, this disease affects as many as one million women, and may cause infertility and tubal (ectopic) pregnancies in about ten percent of infected persons. The bacterium can also grow in the mouth, throat, eyes, and anus. The highest rate of infection is found in women between the ages of fifteen and nineteen and men between the ages of twenty and twenty-four.

http://www.cdc.gov/std/gonorrhea/STDFact-gonorrhea.htm
http://www.niaid.nih.gov/factsheets/stdgon.htm
http://www.health.state.ny.us/nysdoh/communicable_diseases/en/gonor.htm

Herpes

Genital herpes is a sexually transmitted disease (STD) caused by the herpes simplex viruses type 1 (HSV-1) and type 2 (HSV-2). Most genital herpes is caused by HSV-2, although it can also be caused by the HSV-1. Most individuals have no or only minimal signs or symptoms from HSV-1 or HSV-2 infection. When signs do occur, they typically appear as one or more blisters on or around the genitals or rectum. HSV type 1 most commonly infects the lips, causing sores known as fever blisters or cold sores, but it can also infect the genital area and produce sores (also called lesions). The blisters break, leaving tender ulcers (sores) that may take two to four weeks to heal the first time they occur. Typically, another outbreak can appear weeks or months after the first, but it is almost always less severe and shorter than the first outbreak. Although the infection can stay in the body indefinitely, the number of outbreaks tends to decrease over a period of years.

CDC estimates that about forty five million people in the United States, or about twenty percent of the adolescent and adult population, are infected with HSV-2. The largest increase in infection is occurring in young teens.

http://www.cdc.gov/std/Herpes/default.htm
http://www.niaid.nih.gov/factsheets/stdherp.htm
http://www.4woman.gov/faq/stdherpe.htm

Hepatitis B

Hepatitis B is a sexually transmitted disease caused by a virus (HBV) that attacks the liver. The virus is spread through contact with infected blood, sex with an infected person, and from mother to child during childbirth. Although the disease is spread in pretty much the same way as HIV, the Hepatitis B virus is a lot easier to transmit because its concentration in blood is more than a hundred times more than HIV.

Hepatitis B virus can cause scarring of the liver, liver cancer, liver failure, and even death. While there is not yet a cure for HBV the good news is that there is a Hepatitis B vaccine, which is available for people of all ages to prevent the infection.

http://www.cdc.gov/ncidod/diseases/hepatitis/b/
http://digestive.niddk.nih.gov/ddiseases/pubs/viralhepatitis/#hepb
http://www.nfid.org/factsheets/hepbadult.html

HIV/AIDS

HIV, the human immunodeficiency virus, is a virus that kills your body's CD4 cells. CD4 cells (also called T-helper cells) help your body fight off infection and disease. HIV can be passed from person to person if someone with HIV infection has sex with or shares drug injection needles with another person. It also can be passed from a mother to her baby when she is pregnant, when she delivers the baby, or if she breast-feeds her baby.

AIDS, the acquired immunodeficiency syndrome, is a condition you get when HIV destroys your body's immune system. Normally, the body's immune system helps fight off illness. Over time, HIV can weaken the body's immune system to the point that it can no longer fight off infections. When your immune system fails, you can become very sick and can die.

http://www.cdc.gov/hiv/pubs/brochure/atrisk.htm
http://digestive.niddk.nih.gov/ddiseases/pubs/viralhepatitis/#hepb
http://www.nfid.org/factsheets/hepbadult.html

Human Papilloma Virus (HPV)

Human PapillomaVirus (HPV) one of the most common causes of sexually transmitted infections. There are about one hundred different types of HPV. Most of these are harmless, but about thirty types of HPV are transmitted through sexual encounters. HPV infects the genital area of men and women including the skin of the penis, vulva, and anus. HPV may also infect the linings of the vagina, cervix, and rectum.

There are high-risk and low-risk types of HPV. High-risk types of HPV can cause cancer of the cervix, vulva, vagina, and anus in women. Low-risk types may cause genital warts. It may also cause an abnormal Pap smear.

At the time of this writing, it is believed that about twenty million people have this infection, with another five and a half million people being infected annually. On the positive front, clinical trials now in place are assessing the effectiveness of some vaccines to prevent HPV infection.

http://www.cdc.gov/std/HPV/STDFact-HPV.htm
http://www.niaid.nih.gov/factsheets/stdhpv.htm
http://www.vh.org/adult/patient/obgyn/hpvfacts/

Syphilis

Syphilis is a sexually transmitted disease (STD) caused by the bacterium Treponema pallidum. Of great concern is the fact that syphilis infection increases by three to five times the risk of acquiring and transmitting HIV. It is also pertinent to mention that the American College of Obstetricians and Gynecologists reports for the year 1999, the rate of syphilis infection was highest among women between the ages of twenty and twenty-nine. Black women have infection rates that are seven times higher than the female population as a whole.

Syphilis is transmitted from person to person through direct contact with a syphilis sore. Sores occur mainly on the external genitals, vagina, anus, or in the rectum. Sores also can occur on the lips and in the mouth. Transmission of the organism occurs during vaginal, anal, or oral sex. Syphilis cannot be spread through contact with toilet seats, doorknobs, swimming pools, hot tubs, bathtubs, shared clothing, or "by sharing food with an infected person.

Women who are pregnant can pass the disease to their unborn children. Infected children may be born with serious mental and physical health problems. If there is a positive side to this disease, it is the fact that it can be successfully treated and cured.

http://www.niaid.nih.gov/factsheets/stdsyph.htm
http://www.cdc.gov/std/Syphilis/STDFact-Syphilis.htm
http://en.wikipedia.org/wiki/Syphilis

Trichomoniasis

This is another curable sexually transmitted disease. Trichomoniasis infection is caused by a single-celled parasite, *Trichomonas vaginalis*. It is one of the most common sexually transmitted infections, and the Center for Disease Control and Prevention estimates that there are about 7.5 million infections yearly.

Trichomoniasis can be transmitted by both men and women. The vagina is the most common site of infection in women; the disease is usually transmitted by penile intercourse or vulva-to-vulva contact with an infected partner. Although many people have no symptoms, in women, the symptoms can include itching, burning, or irritation in the vagina. These can also be accompanied by yellowish, greenish, or gray discharge from the vagina. Pregnant women with trichomoniasis may have babies who are born early or with low birth weight (less than five pounds).

A pelvic examination in your doctor's office can be used to diagnose the infection. The doctor collects a sample and uses a microscope to look at the specimen to confirm the diagnosis. Treatment of trichmoniasis infection can be effected with a single dose of the drug Metronidazole, which is also safe for use by pregnant women. To avoid re-infection, sex has to be avoided by both partners until completion of treatment.

http://www.cdc.gov/std/trichomoniasis/STDFact-Trichomoniasis.htm
http://www.niaid.nih.gov/factsheets/vaginitis.htm
http://kidshealth.org/parent/infections/std/trichomoniasis XE "trichomoniasis" .html

Other Sexually Transmitted Diseases

Other less common sexually transmitted diseases are listed below. Although they are not discussed here, you are encouraged to seek additional information from your doctor's office or another reliable source and to see your doctor if you believe you may have been exposed to any sexually transmitted disease. You can also get information by surfing to any of the major websites that have been included at the end of this book and searching for information on any of the under-listed sexually transmitted diseases.

Cytomegalovirus
Hepatitis A
Human T-cell lymphotropic virus (HTLV types I and II)
Molluscum contagiosum
Chanchroid
Donovanosis (granuloma inguinale)
Mycoplasma hominis
Nongonococcal urethritis
Shigellosis

Web
Resources

The Internet can be a powerful tool in your quest for knowledge and information about a wide variety of subjects, and we have included a topical list of reputable websites that you may wish to explore. The Internet is a dynamic entity; websites and the information posted within them are constantly changing and evolving. Although we have made every effort to include only accurate current Internet addresses, it is inevitable that some of them may have changed.

Although some links to specific web pages may change, the main websites we have listed are very stable and unlikely to change. If you find that a link to a webpage is broken, you can usually find the information by linking to the home page and using the search tool or site map. For example, if the original link to the website is www.cdc.gov/std/trichomonas and you cannot link to this page, simply truncate the address after the first forward slash (/) and link to the home page, in this case is www.cdc.gov. On the home page, you are likely to find a search box and you will type in the subject, which in this case is trichomoniasis.

Adolescents and Young Adults

TeenSource
www.teensource.org
Created by teens for teens and affiliated with the California Family Health Council, Inc. (CFHC), this site provides resources and information about health and relationship issues affecting teenagers and young adults—both male and female.

KidsHealth
http://kidshealth.org

This award-winning site provides doctor-approved information about children and children's health from pre-birth through adolescence. The site features sections created specifically for parents, children, and teens. Each section includes age-appropriate articles, animations, games, and/or resources created by health care experts.

Powerful Bones, Powerful Girls: The National Bone Health Campaign
http://www.cdc.gov/powerfulbones

This fun site offers information and games that help girls establish nutrition and exercise habits that build and maintain healthy bones.

Nutrition and Weight Management

Centers for Disease Control: Overweight and Obesity Homepage
http://www.cdc.gov/nccdphp/dnpa/obesity

This portion of the CDC site provides information and resources on obesity and weight issues, including definitions, trends, factors, frequently asked questions, resources, and BMI calculator, as well as links to nutrition, physical activity, and other related topics.

American Obesity Association
http://www.obesity.org/

The American Obesity Association (AOA) works to change public policy and perceptions about obesity. The site provides news, information, and advocacy information about obesity.

TeensHealth: Obesity

http://kidshealth.org/teen/food_fitness/dieting/obesity.html

This article for teens describes obesity and its causes and risk factors. It also provides tips and resources for dealing with obesity and weight issues.

Weight-control Information Network

http://win.niddk.nih.gov/

The Weight-Control Information Network (WIN) is a national source of science-based information on weight control, obesity, physical activity, and weight-related nutritional issues for health professionals and the public. The publications section includes articles on topics such as eating disorders, gastric bypass surgery, and healthy weight control.

Surgeon General Topics: Obesity

http://www.surgeongeneral.gov/topics/obesity

Review the Surgeon General's "Call to Action" press release, download fact sheets, or link to resources about obesity and nutrition.

WebMD Health Guide: Gastric Bypass

http://www.webmd.com/hw/weight_control/hw252819.asp

This article on WebMD provides a comprehensive overview of gastric bypass surgery, including illustrations and links to additional resources and related topics.

healthfinder,: Obesity

http://www.healthfinder.gov/scripts/SearchContext.asp?topic=592

This page in healthfinder.com links to health news and resources about obesity, nutrition, treatment, and weight control.

Cancer

Gynecologic Cancer Foundatiion

http://www.thegcf.org

The mission of the Gynecologic Cancer Foundation (GCF) is to ensure public awareness of gynecologic cancer prevention, early diagnosis and proper treatment as well as supports research and training related to gynecologic cancers. This website provides the report "State of the State of Gynecologic Cancers: Third Annual Report to the Women of America."

Susan G. Komen Breast Cancer Foundation

http://www.komen.org

The Komen foundation supports breast cancer research and community-based outreach programs for education, screening, and treatment. The site also provides information and links about breast cancer, as well as a breast cancer helpline.

Breastcancer.org

http://www.breastcancer.org

The mission of breastcancer.org is to provide accurate, up-to-date, and easily understandable medical information. Features of the site include research news, pictures of breast cancer, and monthly online ask-the-expert conferences, as well as discussion boards and chat rooms for anyone affected by breast cancer.

National Cancer Institute

http://www.cancer.gov

This site from the U.S. Institutes of Health offers information about a number of topics related to all types of cancer, including breast cancer. Specific information regarding treatment, prevention, screening, and clinical trials is provided for each cancer topic, as well as additional resources for those coping with or seeking treatment for cancer.

American Institute for Cancer Research (AICR)
http://www.aicr.org

AICR is a cancer charity that supports research and education on the role of diet and nutrition in the treatment and prevention of cancer. The site features the AICR's Diet and Health Guidelines for Cancer Prevention, as well as educational information, news, recipes, and a nutrition hotline.

American Cancer Society
http://www.cancer.org

The American Cancer Society is a nationwide, community-based organization whose focus is to eliminate cancer. The ACS website offers medical information, treatment decision tools, news updates, support resources, and stories of hope for cancer patients and survivors as well as family, friends, and health professionals. The site also provides community-based information and links to volunteer and advocacy opportunities.

Substance Abuse

National Clearinghouse for Alcohol and Drug Information (NCADI)
http://www.health.org

The National Clearinghouse for Alcohol and Drug Information (NCADI) is designed as a one-stop resource for information about substance abuse prevention and addiction treatment. The site offers links to resources as well as free or low-cost publications from a wide variety of government agencies and non-profit organizations. Materials can be downloaded or ordered online.

National Institute on Alcohol Abuse and Alcoholism (NIAAA)
http://www.niaaa.nih.gov

The NIAAA website offers resources, information, and publications related to understanding, treating, and preventing alcohol abuse.

National Institute on Drug Abuse (NIDA)

http://www.drugabuse.gov

The mission of NIDA is to bring the power of science to bear on drug abuse and recovery. Their website offers educational resources and materials for students and young adults; drug facts, information, and educational materials for parents and teachers; and links to NIDA sites on specific drugs and issues.

Mental Health

National Institutes of Mental Health (NIMH)

http://www.nimh.nih.gov

The NIMH website features health information and coverage of breaking news and research in the area of mental health.

About.com: Mental Health

http://mentalhealth.about.com

This section of About.com includes mental health resources, articles, essential information, and answers to common questions about mental health issues and conditions.

National Alliance on Mental Illness (NAMI)

http://www.nami.org

NAMI is the United States' largest grassroots mental health organization dedicated to improving the lives of persons living with mental illness and their families. The site provides content about illnesses, medications, and current research, as well as links to additional resources for information and support. The site also includes sections on advocacy, policy, and action.

Comprehensive Health-related Websites

Agency for Healthcare Research and Quality (AHRQ)
http://www.ahrq.gov

This agency of the U.S. Department of Health and Human Services (HHS) supports research and provides information aimed at helping people make better decisions about health care. The Consumers & Patients section includes information and resources that help visitors to the site become more active in their own healthcare.

WomensHealth.gov
http://www.womenshealth.gov

This is the website of the National Women's Health Information Center (NWHIC). The website offers information on more than 800 topics, including pregnancy, breastfeeding, body image, HIV/AIDS, girls health, heart health, menopause and hormone therapy, mental health, quitting smoking, and violence against women.

U.S. Centers for Disease Control (CDC)
http://www.cdc.gov

The CDC website is continually updated with feature articles addressing current health topics and issues. The site also provides a wide array of topical health and safety information, data and statistics, and access to health-related publications and products

healthfinder®
http://www.healthfinder.gov

Developed by the U.S. Department of Health and Human Services, healthfinder is an easy-to-use guide to reliable health information. The library section offers information on prevention and wellness, diseases and conditions, and alternative medicine, as well as medical dictionaries and encyclopedia. The site also provides health news, a directory of organizations, and more than 50 "Online Checkups."

American College of Obstetricians and Gynecologists (ACOG)

http://www.acog.org

This site for members of the ACOG also offers "Find an Ob-Gyn," an online locater service to help you found a doctor in your area.

Medline Plus

http://www.medlineplus.gov

Medline Plus offers extensive information and resources on health topics. Search the site for answers to health questions or browse the list of health topics. Medline Plus also has extensive information about drugs, an illustrated medical encyclopedia, interactive patient tutorials, and current health news.

Familydoctor.org

http://www.familydoctor.org

This site from the American Academy of Family Physicians features "Conditions A to Z," a searchable collection of articles on many common conditions and health concerns. Specific pages address health specific topics for women, kids, men, and seniors. Special sections offer a Smart Patient Guide, Healthy Living information, a guide to over-the-counter medicines, and tools such as a medical dictionary.

HIV InSite

http://hivinsite.org

HIV InSite is developed by the Center for HIV Information (CHI) at the University of California San Francisco (UCSF). The site includes extensive information about HIV/AIDs care, prevention, treatment, and policy in the United States and around the world. Also included are links to many other online resources, including the Women, Children, and HIV website, and a question and answer feature.

Mayo Clinic

http://www.mayoclinic.org

The Mayo Clinic offers an alphabetical index of diseases, treat-
ments, and services for patients (and non-patients), along with
"Medical Edge" health stories, health news, and information on
clinical trials.

Medem

http://medem.com/MedLB/medlib_entry.cfm

http://medem.com/pat/pat.cfm

Medem is a physician-patient communications network that
includes over 90,000 physicians. The Patients section features an
online medical library, a doctor finder service, and the Smart
Parents' Health Source newsletter. You can also create a confiden-
tial iHealthRecord, where you can store, update, and share health
information with your physician

New York Online Access to Health (NOAH)

http://www.noah-health.org

NOAH provides access to quality-filtered consumer health information. The information is selected and screened by librarians
and health professionals to ensure that it is current, accurate, and
unbiased. Sections include health topics listed by disease category
or body area, an alphabetic index, and a featured page of the
month.

American Medical Association (AMA)

http://www.ama-assn.org

The website of the American Medical Association offers a doctor
finder feature as well as health news and information on healthcare advocacy issues supported by the association.

American Heart Association
http://www.americanheart.org

The American Heart Association works to reduce disability and death from cardiovascular diseases and stroke. The website offers a wealth of information and resources on preventing and treating heart disease, maintaining healthy lifestyles, and even children's health.

WebMD
http://www.webmd.com

WebMD provides credible health information, tools for managing your health, and support for those who seek information. The section on diseases and conditions includes an A–Z guide, specific information for men and women, and an interactive "Check Your Symptoms" feature. Other features include guidance for health-care services, resources for pregnancy and family, and various message boards and blogs.

Reproductive Health Outlook (RHO)
http://www.rho.org

RHO is a project of Program for Appropriate Technology in Health (PATH), an international, nonprofit organization that creates sustainable, culturally relevant solutions, enabling communities worldwide to break longstanding cycles of poor health. The RHO website provides in-depth information on reproductive health and links to online resources for additional information.

National Women's Health Resource Center (NWHRC)
http://www.healthywomen.org

The National Women's Health Resource Center is dedicated to helping women make informed decisions about their health and embrace healthy lifestyles to promote wellness and prevent disease. The website provides access to comprehensive health information from medical and health experts.

Additional Websites of Interest

Village.com

http://www.ivillage.com

iVillage is an online network for women. Sections on health, beauty, diet and fitness, and pregnancy and parenting feature articles, expert advice, newsletters, and message boards. The site also includes links to women's magazines such as Cosmopolitan, Redbook, and Marie Claire.

Oprah.com

http://www.oprah.com

Read features related to the Oprah show and visit sections on health, well-being, relationships, and the Angel Network.

Essence

http://www.essence.com

The website for Essence Magazine includes online features, links, and a monthly newsletter for the latest beauty, fashion and entertainment news, and events.

Real Simple

http://www.realsimple.com

This website as its names suggests provides ideas on how to make life easier. It offers numerous tips on organizing, meals, cleaning, and life skills, all with a view of simplifying our lives.

Every Woman

http://www.everywomanonline.com

Every Woman is a bilingual, multimedia women's healthcare brand from the. The Association of Women's Health and Neonatal Nurses. The site provides downloadable versions of articles from its publications in both Spanish and English

Glamour: Health & Body

http://www.glamour.com/health

This section of Glamour magazine's website includes articles and features related to women's health.

About.com: Women's Health

http://womenshealth.about.com

About.com's section on women's health features articles, resources, and links to health-related online offers.

Ortho Women's Health

http://www.orthowomenshealth.com

This website is operated by Ortho-McNeil Pharmaceutical, Inc. and covers various aspects of women's health including, but not limited to birth control, gynecological health, migraine, and bladder health. This website also has an excellent webpage on how to prepare for a visit to your doctor.

Epilogue

Who are my sisters? If you are a woman, you are my sister. You are my sister, regardless of class or color, race or religion. You are my sister as long as you love me as you love yourself. Our commonalities are much more than our differences, and the conditions that affect us do not discriminate, whether we are in high places or reside in slums. The stressors in our lives are the same, even if the degrees to which they affect us are different. The symptoms of urinary tract infections are the same for all women, whether you are a millionaire heiress or a pauper.

An investment for you is truly the best thing. Apologies to Martha Stewart - it is a good thing. What kind of investment am I writing about? I am referring to investment in your health. How do you get about making the investment? You do so by exercising the body, stimulating the mind, and uplifting the spirit. It truly is the best insurance policy for protecting oneself against the vagaries of aging. It is especially important during these times with the inflationary trend of the cost of healthcare. It is well documented that the quality of life as we mature greatly depends on how we have treated ourselves at a younger age. Good habits are very difficult to form, but a lot easier when we are younger. Let us do the right things now to minimize the potential of spending half our pensions on medicines, or worse still, having to decide between medicines and food during the sunset years. To the extent that we know that an active and healthy lifestyle reduces the chance of some forms of illness, as we get older, it reinforces the need to start early.

It is never too early to start healthy habits, nor is it ever too late. Resolve to make the necessary changes, even if it means starting from a series of small steps. A journey of a thousand miles starts with a step. Make that move today. Begin the journey on the route to a healthier you. Create positive change. Eat better. Exercise regularly. Encourage other sisters. Love a lot. Smile. Read. Write. Crotchet. Knit. Volunteer. Do a 5K walk. A 10K run. Run or walk a marathon with a relay team of sisters, and maybe brothers, too. Donate time. Contribute money. Don't worry. Be happy.

My life has been enriched by the interactions I have had with all my sisters. I have cried on the shoulders of some, I have laughed with others, and I have strived with others to get to where I am today. As I mentioned in the prologue, this book started out as a way of giving back to my sisters, who were also my patients. The people who got an early peek of the manuscript felt that the contents should be shared by every woman and encouraged me to have it published for a wider audience. I hope this book gives back something to all of you, some of whom I have met personally, some of whom I have read about, and others still, who have impacted my life by their words in print and electronic media. If you feel I have been overly blunt, forgive me, because that's what sisters do. I have some flaws like most people, although I strive to improve, but sisters always accept sisters, warts and all. May the Almighty bless and reward you for all that you do take care of his temple and to improve humanity.

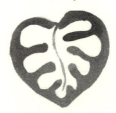

Notes on Sources

The poem 'The One in the Glass' was retrieved from a promotional material developed by Clark, Schaefer, Hackett and Company, a certified public accounting and business consultancy firm in Ohio.

In this book, the quotes used have been selected from a variety of books and websites on the Internet. The majority of the quotes came from the books listed below, in no particular order:

Biggs, Mary. *Women's Words: The Columbia Book of Quotation by Women*. Columbia University Press, New York, 1996.

Hewlett, Rasheen. *Pearls of Black Wisdom*
Peter Pauper Press, Inc., White Plains, New York, 1999

Quinn, Tracy. *Quotable Women of the Twentieth Century*
William Morrow and Company, Inc., New York 1999.

Murphy, Edward F. Murphy. *2,715 One-Line Quotations for Speakers, Writers and Raconteurs*, Gramercy Books, New York, 1996.

Frank, Leonard Roy. *Random House Webster's Quotationary: The authoritative source for 20000 quotations*. Random House, New York 2001

Partnow, Elaine Bernstein. *The Quotable Jewish Woman: Wisdom, Inspiration and Humor from the Mind and Heart*. Jewish Lights Publishing, Woodstock, Vermont, 2004.

Lovric, Michelle. *Women's Wicked Wit: from Jane Austen to Roseanne Barr.*
North American Edition, Chicago Review Press, 2001.

The quote by Catherine Pulsifer was obtained from the website: http://www.stresslesscountry.com/lifestyle-quotes.
The quotes by Pam Brown and Barbara Alpert were obtained from the website: http://www.quotegarden.com/sisters.html

In writing this book, multiple websites were reviewed and efforts were made to acknowledge them after each topic discussed in the second part of the book. In addition to the websites, these two publications listed below were also consulted in writing this book. The Pocket Guide to Good Health for Adults provides some very useful tit-bits and can be obtained free from AHQR. The Women's Health Stats and Facts 2004 Pocket Guide from ACOG is an excellent source for statistical information on women's health.

Agency for Healthcare Research and Quality. *The Pocket Guide to Good Health for Adults*. U.S. Department of Health and Human Services. 2003.

The American College of Obstetricians and Gynecologists. *Women's Health. Stats and Facts. 2004 Pocket Guide*. ACOG, Washington D.C., 2005.

Index

Give the Gift of Caring

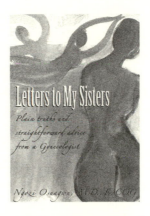

This book is available at Amazon, Barnes and Nobles,
Booksense® Stores, or wherever books are sold.
Copies of the book can also be purchased directly from Ben Bosah Books.
Phone Sales: (614) 939-0595
or on the Internet at www.letterstomysisters.com
or write us at Ben Bosah Books, P O Box 671, New Albany, Ohio 43054.

Ben Bosah Books will make copies of Letters to My Sisters available at
special quantity discounts for bulk purchases for sales promotions, premiums, fund-
raising, health fairs, or educational use. Special books or books excerpts can also be
created from Letters to My Sisters to suit specific requirements.

Order forms can be downloaded from http://www.letterstomysisters.com
or copied from the back of this page.

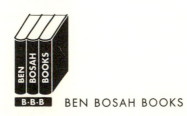

BEN BOSAH BOOKS

ORDER FORM

(1-10 COPIES)

Payable in United States funds only. Price per book: $16.95
Postage and handling: $4.00 for one book, $1.00 each additional book,
not to exceed $10.00. We accept bank checks, money orders and credit cards.
Please do not send cash. We do not accept cash on delivery (COD).
Allow 2 to 4 weeks for delivery, unless requesting expedited delivery.

Call (614) 939-0595 or fax orders to (614) 939-0596, or mail your orders to:
Ben Bosah Books, P O Box 671, New Albany, Ohio 43054.

NAME _____

COMPANY _____

ADDRESS _____

_____

CITY _____ STATE _____ ZIP _____

TELEPHONE (DAYTIME) _____

CREDIT CARD ☐ VISA ☐ MASTERCARD ☐ AMERICAN EXPRESS

CREDIT CARD NUMBER _____

SIGNATURE _____

QUANTITY OF BOOKS _____

BOOK TOTAL _____

SALES TAX _____

SHIPPING AND HANDLING _____

TOTAL _____

SHIP TO:

NAME _____

COMPANY _____

ADDRESS _____

_____

CITY _____ STATE _____ ZIP _____